feel-good fitness

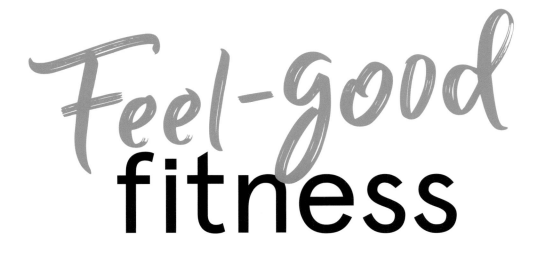

Feel-good fitness

FUN WORKOUT CHALLENGES TO INSPIRE YOUR FITNESS STREAK

Alysia Montaño

VELO PRESS

Boulder, Colorado

To my mom and dad, Yvonne and Eric; my big brother, Eric II (the cinnamon-stick head to my apple head); my cousins (my best friends); and my aunts and uncles (the village). To Louis—my husband, my ride or die, my partner and biggest supporter, my right hand. And of course to the family that we call our own—Linnéa, Aster, and Lennox . . . my babies.

▼velopress®

4745 Walnut Street, Unit A
Boulder, CO 80301-2587 USA

VeloPress is the leading publisher of books on endurance sports and is a division of Pocket Outdoor Media. Focused on cycling, triathlon, running, swimming, and nutrition/diet, VeloPress books help athletes achieve their goals of going faster and farther. Preview books and contact us at velopress.com.

Distributed in the United States and Canada by Ingram Publisher Services

Library of Congress Cataloging-in-Publication Data
Names: Montaño, Alysia, author.
Title: Feel-good fitness: fun workout challenges to inspire your fitness
    streak / Alysia Montaño.
Description: Boulder, Colorado: VeloPress, [2020]
Identifiers: LCCN 2019058089 (print) | LCCN 2019058090 (ebook) | ISBN
    9781948007030 (paperback) | ISBN 9781948006194 (ebook)
Subjects: LCSH: Physical fitness. | Running.
Classification: LCC GV481 .M626 2020 (print) | LCC GV481 (ebook) | DDC
    613.7—dc23
LC record available at https://lccn.loc.gov/2019058089
LC ebook record available at https://lccn.loc.gov/2019058090

This paper meets the requirements of ANSI/NISO Z39.48-1992
(Permanence of Paper).

Art direction and interior design by Vicki Hopewell
Cover and interior photos by Jeff Clark / Pixel Peak
Cover design by Megan Roy

20 21 22 / 10 9 8 7 6 5 4 3 2 1

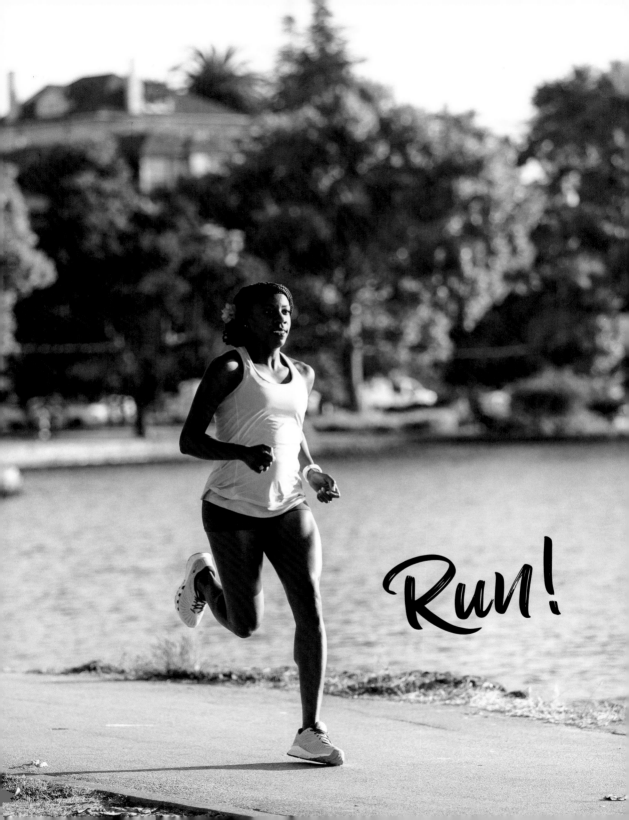

Run!

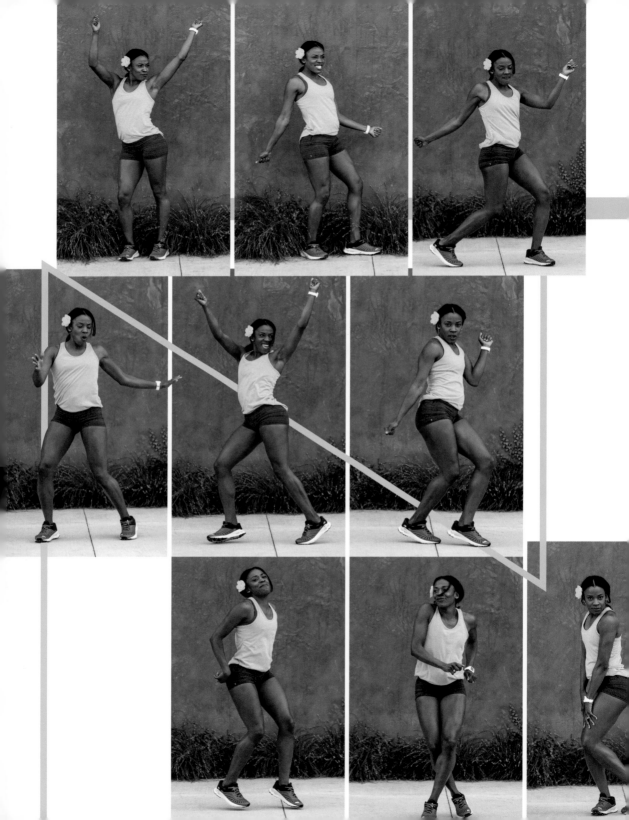

Challenges

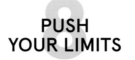
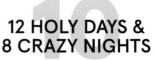

Your fitness streak starts here

In my experience, most of us know we should work out, and many of us even want to work out, but we have no idea where or how to begin. *What if I don't belong to a gym? But I don't have much time!* I guarantee that if you can start a program and stick to it, you will begin to want more. Fitness doesn't need to be a burden. Done right, a healthy, fit lifestyle doesn't have to cost a lot or put you in a pain cave . . . being fit can feel good!

As a mother and an athlete, I want to be better and I recognize that means I need to "practice" every single day. I want to model for my kids what it looks like to be fierce and resilient. Now, I'll be the first to admit I am human and, like anyone, my motivation can wane, but I know that if I can get one foot out the door the other will quickly follow and my children will see that mama also has rough days but she doesn't give up. I know that once I get

started I will start to feel better. On days when it is just straight torture, I think about how much better I will feel having fought through a mentally tough day. Barring sickness, exercise is a great mood booster. Once you start sweating, those endorphins start working their magic.

Your body wants to work for you. It's time to begin thinking about how you move through everyday life, and commit to moving your body so you can be better.

Fitness is a great metaphor for life. It is a space to challenge yourself, to reach a goal, to hit a PR, and to progress in ways big and small. Whether you want to become a better runner or just start running, the big idea here is growth. Let's not settle for more of the same. If you have reached a plateau physically or emotionally, let's take on a new challenge and see what happens.

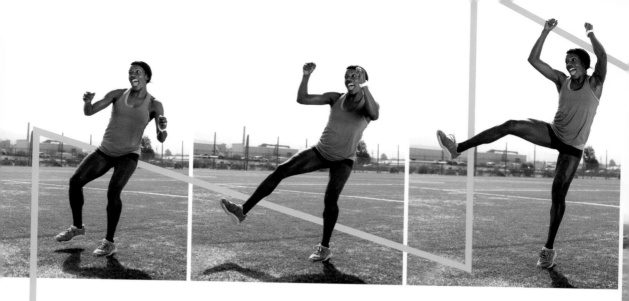

But I'm not a runner!

I may be an Olympic middle-distance runner, but I wasn't born with a passion for running. What I did have right from the start was passion to move, to push myself, to feel the adrenaline. I always enjoyed being able to take on a challenge, and figure out ways to become better, to overcome weaknesses, and get after my goals. Through this process I developed a hard-core passion for movement. I love how movement helps me carry on through my daily life with energy and pride. I love how movement also shows me that I am strong, I am resilient, and I have the tremendous ability to persevere and to overcome obstacles. I have the ability to take a challenge head-on, knowing it isn't going to be easy, but knowing the hard-fought effort is worth it.

The great thing about running is that it is so accessible. Find yourself a good pair of shoes, a watch, and a foam roller, and you are all good. Run repeatedly and you just might start to feel truly free, like you can fly. It's not a speed thing; it's all about moving athletically, and all of the "feels" that come with that.

Move better, run better

In track and field, we spend a lot of time working on agility and quickness. Activation drills and strength training play a huge role in the training and preparation of professional athletes, and I credit this work with keeping me relatively

USE WHAT YOU'VE GOT! Everyday items like countertops, beds, couches, desks, window ledges, and sturdy chairs double as awesome, immensely practical exercise benches. Knocking out some incline push-ups? Grab a surface that's at the height you need, and get to it!

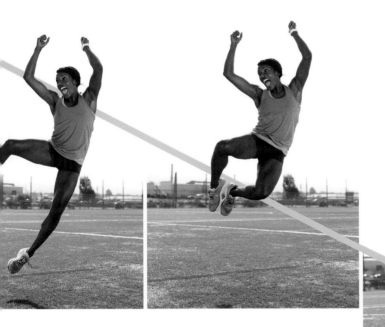

injury-free. Among distance and recreational runners, this kind of work is often overlooked in favor of higher miles. I regularly encounter runners who tell me that they don't spend time in the weight room. Running puts forces on your body that pack a punch—almost three times your body weight. What makes us think that we don't need to pick up a weight, use a band, or do the work that will make us better runners? If you want to improve efficiency, speed, and endurance, if you want to run stronger and farther, this is an investment you can take to the bank. Do the work and you can build from a place of balance, rather than waiting for the chain to break and then trying to get back to balance.

Even now, most of the workouts I do entail activation drills. After all, we need to prepare our bodies to move. Imagine your morning without a coffee, or being woken up and immediately expected to perform at your best. Warming up prior to a workout, doing activation drills, is like communicating to your body, "We are about to do a little bit more, you cool?" Get it done and you can hear your body say, "Yeah, let's do this."

You need your body to work with you, not against you. Naturally, your body will move better when it's warm. Temperature matters—a cold rubber band can snap if you don't take the time to warm it up and restore its elasticity. Treat your body to a warm-up every time you work out.

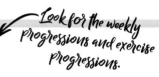
Look for the weekly progressions and exercise progressions.

WEEKLY PROGRESSIONS (SAMPLE)
Week 2: Progress Superwoman to Twisting Superwoman
Week 3: Progress Mountain Climber to Twisting Mountain Climber

Sometimes an individual exercise will have an option:
≪ To make it easier   ≫ To make it harder

This makes it easy to challenge yourself week over week.

After the warm-up, activation drills teach your body to fire optimally to avoid injury. It's easy to lose sight of this, but if you show your body how to move in an efficient way, you will fire up the neurological pathways that put peak performance on autopilot. Put in this time and you will find it easier to move athletically and over time you can expect more from your body.

Pick a challenge

I've mapped out 10 challenges for you, but don't feel like you have to tackle them in order. If you haven't been running or working out regularly, Challenge 1 is a great place to start. Whatever you do, find a challenge that you are excited about and get after it. On the back half, the challenges will progress strength and speed work in new ways.

I've designed these challenges to make fitness more attainable for all of us. Here's what you can expect:

Workouts that fit your life. Most are 30 minutes or less. Each challenge has 4–6

workouts that you can fit into your week on the days that work best for you. Pick your own recovery days.

Variety, but not too much of it. If you are doing a 4-week challenge you will repeat the weekly workouts four times. There's just enough repetition to build confidence and just enough variety to keep you from getting bored. Just look for the weekly progressions and exercise progressions so you can keep challenging yourself along the way.

A finish line that you can reach. Too many times we start an ambitious training program or join a gym and after a while we lose motivation. My challenges are just 2–4 weeks in duration. Why? Because we all need to feel validated by reaching our goal.

How to navigate pace and effort

If you've been running for years, you might know how fast you can run a mile or a 5K. If you've only run when someone was chasing you, I've got your back. I like

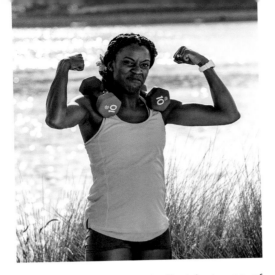

to talk about pace and effort in terms of how it feels. After all, I want you to listen to your body every step of the way. So, as you run, gauge perceived effort on a scale of 1–10. In the RPE chart below you will see a description of effort levels and the running paces that typically correlate with them.

If you train with a watch, you will begin to figure out what your typical pace is at different distances over time. I've also added in some of the different run paces used throughout the challenges that follow so you can know what to expect. We will also do some benchmark tests and time trials to give you a better sense of how to pace your workouts.

One important thing to keep in mind is that the same pace can feel really different from one day to the next. If you didn't sleep well or if stress has you at the max before you even put your shoes on, chances are good that a hard effort will feel even harder. This is why it's important to listen to your body. Give it your best, but stay true to how the effort should feel, trusting that you'll have another chance at busting out that top speed.

What if I miss a workout?

I'll just call it right now. You will miss some workouts. Whether you get sucked into a big deadline at work, get sick, find yourself taking care of your kids, oversleep, undersleep, or experience any

RPE	1	2	3	4	5
		COOLDOWN	WARM-UP	LONG + SLOW	STEADY-STATE
	Yo, is that all you got?	This feels chill.	Warming up and loving it.	Feeling the rhythm.	Is it getting hot in here?
	6	7	8	9	10
	TEMPO	THRESHOLD, HILLS	SPEED + POWER	SPRINT	
	Heart is thumping and I've got less to say.	This is getting harder.	Don't even talk to me.	Giving it everything I've got.	Please stop me from dialing the 1 for 9-1- . . .

other insurmountable obstacle in a day, let's just accept that it will happen and move on.

The whole point of setting a fitness streak is to know what it feels like to consistently make time for moving and feeling good. Do it and you'll want more of it. So stop beating yourself up over a missed workout. Tomorrow's a new day. Commit to your workout and get back on track.

Balance work and recovery

You'll notice that every challenge includes recovery days. You can either take the day off or do some active recovery work—get out your foam roller or do some light mobility work.

I like to take the weekends off so I have more time with my family. Lots of people like to do longer workouts on the weekends, but I prefer to be home rolling my glutes out while the kids do their weekend thing instead of trying to make the morning revolve around my workout. You might want to pace your longer ones throughout the week or get up super early. Do what works best for you, but find your off switch.

Fitness works when you fit it in around the parts of your life that fulfill you. Remember to ask for help in balancing all of the responsibilities a week holds—work, laundry, wiping butts, making meals. You'll have more energy for all of that when you get back from your workout.

Show up ready

Food, water, and rest will help you get the best from your body. I go out of my way to eat healthy, organic foods because I feel better when I fuel better. Maybe there are some small steps you can take to eat and fuel better. With each challenge, try to introduce one small change. It gets easier to make good choices when you feel the difference it makes.

Prior to working out, I like to eat a Picky Bar. In my experience, even half of a bar in my belly 30 minutes prior to working out is better than nothing. Find what works best for you—every body is different. Have a snack ready after working out.

WORKOUT TERMINOLOGY	CIRCUITS	SUPERSETS
Here are some guidelines to help you make sense of the workouts.	A circuit is a series of exercises to be repeated. For example, you might do 5 exercises, rest 30 seconds, and then repeat those 5 exercises for a total of three rounds, or three times. Each exercise in a circuit is numbered. *Like this* →1	A superset is a smaller set of complimentary exercises that you repeat until you have completed the number of rounds specified. There is often a short rest between rounds. Each superset is numbered. *Like this* →1

We are less likely to crave unhealthy foods or binge eat if we can refuel at the right times. If you're reaching for a doughnut after your workout, you probably didn't refuel right. There's nothing that doughnut is giving back to your body. Listen, there's a time for doughnuts, but make sure you refuel right.

Remember to hydrate before, during, and after exercise. How you hydrate depends on the workout, but here are some simple tricks:

▸ Invest in a 24-ounce water bottle that you can carry with you throughout the day.
▸ Plan on drinking at least 8–16 ounces before you exercise.
▸ As you work out, rehydrate between intervals or sets—sips, not gulps are best to make sure you don't end up with stomach cramps.
▸ Include electrolytes in at least one water bottle during exercise to replace the minerals that you lose when you sweat.

▸ Be deliberate about drinking liquids immediately after exercise.

On recovery days, remember to think about hydration. For me, a typical day off includes plenty of Nuun Rest with magnesium and tart cherry, which aids in sleep and recovery.

Get your head in the game

Whenever I'm physically working, I also want to be mentally working. When mind and body work together, the hard work of training can take full effect and we can be more prepared for anything life throws at us.

With each challenge, I've sprinkled in some *Flower Power*—these are attributes that deserve our attention because they have the power to change how we think about ourselves and what we can do. Promise me you will make some space to think about these things—you owe it to yourself.

Enough talk. Let's do this!

REPS

The number of repetitions for a given exercise. If it's a bilateral exercise (working each side separately), do the full rep count on each side. If it's an alternating movement, you will move left and right to count one rep. There are a few exercises where we will work each side separately and also change direction halfway through the rep count. Don't worry, I'll remind you.

AMRAP (As Many Reps As Possible)

Get the rep count as high as you can while still keeping your form intact. Don't try to be a hero and go to failure on these. I want you to be able to move when chased by a predator. Those last 3 reps are no good if you can't run for your life.

TIMED INTERVALS

Rather than providing a rep count, some workouts will specify a timed interval for each exercise.

Challenge 1

KICK-START YOUR RUNNING RESOLUTION

If you want to build a running habit you love, this is the perfect place to start! As you might have experienced in the past, when taking on a new challenge, the tiniest of things can turn into major deterrents. The most common one? Trying to do too much right away.

I know, I know—you're excited to give your running resolution all you've got, and I'm telling you to slow your roll. But hear me out: When you go from 0 to 60 in a single day, you're pretty much guaranteed to burn out just as fast.

After all, rocking this challenge might sound like a single to-do, but in reality, it could involve a dozen or more. Maybe you need to buy running shoes, wake up earlier, find someone to watch your kiddos, adjust your nutrition to support your workouts, get comfortable with delayed onset muscle soreness (DOMS), create the perfect running playlist; the list goes on and adds up fast.

This challenge is all about keeping to-dos (those pesky deterrents) to a minimum and setting you up for running-resolution success. Each week, you'll perform five short workouts on the days that work for you. All you'll need are running shoes and 20 to 30 minutes to get it done.

Together, your workouts will give you the running foundation you'll need for future challenges. You'll learn the fundamentals of running, in a fun, engaging way so you don't have to risk workout-wrecking boredom. We'll celebrate your progress along the way and build the momentum you need to make running an empowering, lifelong habit.

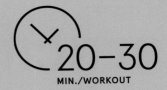

20–30
MIN./WORKOUT

5 days per week for *4 weeks*

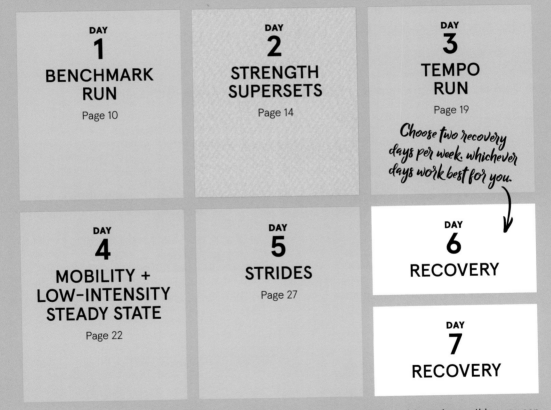

DAY **1** BENCHMARK RUN Page 10	**DAY** **2** STRENGTH SUPERSETS Page 14	**DAY** **3** TEMPO RUN Page 19
DAY **4** MOBILITY + LOW-INTENSITY STEADY STATE Page 22	**DAY** **5** STRIDES Page 27	**DAY** **6** RECOVERY
		DAY **7** RECOVERY

Choose two recovery days per week, whichever days work best for you.

RECOVERY DAYS You don't *have* to work out on recovery days, but if consistency is your thing, you can do the **Foam Rolling** and **Mobility** routines in the Appendix (p. 270) to feel refreshed and ready to crush your workouts ahead. Also, keep in mind that recovery doesn't have to happen at the end of your week. Listen to your body and work recovery days into your schedule when you need them!

EQUIPMENT Running shoes

BENCHMARK RUN

Start each week off by checking in with yourself! This workout will take you through a gentle warm-up, activation drills, and a 1-mile max time trial. Track your results from week to week to celebrate your progress.

WARM-UP

▶ Complete an easy 5-minute walk-jog to get your heart rate up and muscles ready to go. Aim for an average RPE of 3 to 4.

ACTIVATION DRILLS

▶ Do 6 reps of each exercise, resting 15 seconds between each exercise.

DONKEY KICK

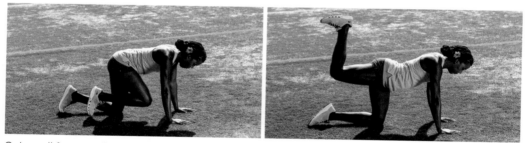

Get on all fours, and engage your glutes to raise your foot up behind you and lower it back down with control. Use your core to keep your back flat and feel the glutes burn, even on the stationary leg. Work both sides.

FIRE HYDRANT

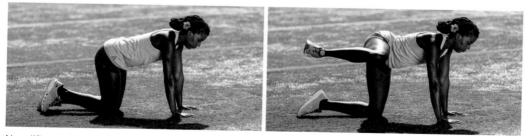

Now lift one leg out laterally and lower it with control. Work both sides.

DEAD BUG

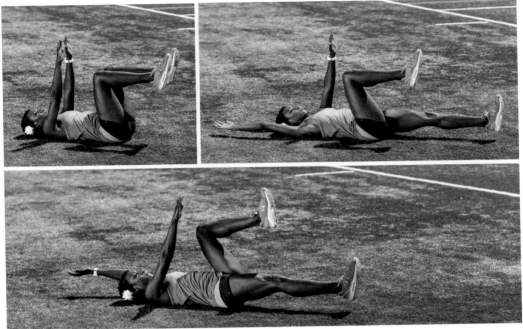

Get set with your low back flat on the ground, arms extended up, knees bent. Move your opposing arm and leg to reach long while you move the opposite hand toward your knee. Keep alternating the movement, slow and controlled.

Goal setting

I'm sure you have heard the saying: "Failing to plan is planning to fail." This proves to be true when it comes to putting together a fitness streak. I've given you a plan for what needs to happen. It's up to you to figure out what might stand in the way of you executing on that plan—work, parenthood, the daily grind. Own this part of the plan and back it up with a contingency plan.

Once your plan is in place, take the opportunity to speak your goal into existence. There is real power to be had in doing this simple thing before you get to work on manifesting it. It's like a promise you make to yourself: it creates accountability and lights a fire in your belly. You owe it to yourself to keep your word and answer the challenge.

A-SKIP

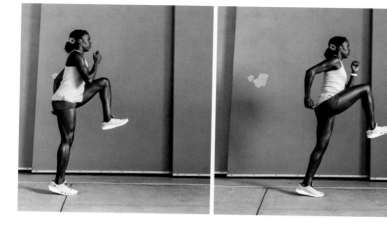

Hop-skip with high knees, swinging your arms to keep momentum.

HIGH KNEES

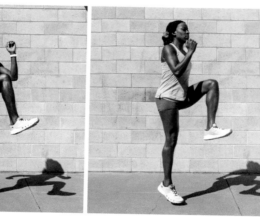

Drive one knee up, and feel the lift as you hop-skip up to the ball of your foot; alternate sides. Drive your arms in a tight stride, opposite your legs. This is a quick, stationary movement.

RUN

TIME TRIAL Give it all you've got! Using a running watch or following a set 1-mile course, time how fast you can run 1 mile (RPE 8).

WEEKLY PROGRESSIONS
Your time trial will feel just as hard from week to week, but that's okay! You will likely be able to shave a few seconds off your time as you get stronger, faster, and more confident!

▶ Hold each stretch for 5 seconds, take a breath, and see if you can stretch a little farther. Do this 5–6 times, then repeat on the other side.

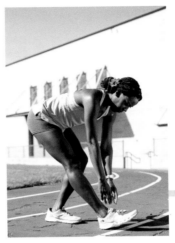

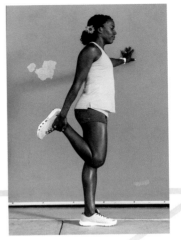

STANDING HAMSTRING STRETCH

Extend one leg just out in front of you and let the knee of the opposite leg bend as you reach forward. Try to keep your back flat.

STANDING QUAD STRETCH

Using a wall for support, stand on one leg and pull the opposite heel to your glute. Press forward through your stretched side to keep your hips and knees square.

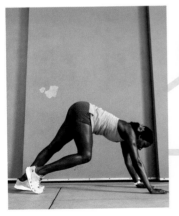

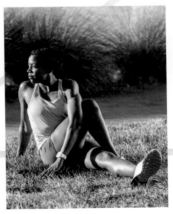

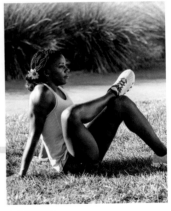

DOWNWARD DOG CALF STRETCH

Push your palms and heels into the ground, bending one knee at a time as you push the opposite heel to the ground to stretch that calf.

SEATED SPINAL ROTATION

With legs extended, cross one leg over the other and twist in the opposite direction, using your arm to push your knee in toward your chest.

SEATED GLUTE STRETCH

With knees bent, cross one leg over the other to get into a figure-4 position. Gently move closer to your stationary foot to intensify the stretch.

STRENGTH SUPERSETS

Some runners love to avoid strength training in favor of more runs, but not us! This body-weight strength workout operates as a circuit to keep you moving, prevent boredom, increase bone density, and improve your cardio too.

▶ **Perform the supersets by doing 8 to 12 reps of each exercise. Rest for 1 minute; then repeat the superset for a total of three rounds. Do this for each superset.**

WEEKLY PROGRESSIONS
Week 2: Use a 2:1:1 tempo.
Week 3: Use a 2:1:1 tempo. Reduce rest between rounds to 30 seconds.
Week 4: Use a 2:1:1 tempo. Maintain rest between rounds at 30 seconds. Boost rep count to 12 to 14 reps, which is when you feel like you can't perform one more rep.

Count your tempo!

Tempo work—timing how long you perform the different phases of any given exercise—is a great way to make those exercises much harder, but without needing to tack on more reps and sets or use more weight. This is especially handy when you're working with your body weight and can't just grab a heavier dumbbell.

Tempos are expressed in seconds as eccentric:pause:concentric. The eccentric phase is the "easy" part of the exercise, the pause happens between the two parts, and the concentric phase is the "hard" part, which happens when you're really putting in the effort.

In body-weight exercises, what you're really fighting against is gravity. That means that the lowering phase is always eccentric and the lifting phase is always concentric. So, when you do a body-weight squat with a 2:1:1 tempo, you'll lower over the course of two seconds, pause for one, and explosively press back up to start in one second. Much tougher, right?

1 BODY-WEIGHT SQUAT

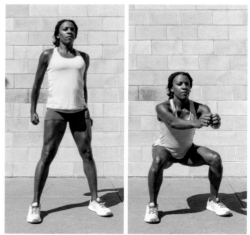

Squat down until your hips and knees are level; then stand back up straight. Whenever you squat, sit back to keep from placing strain on your knees.

INCLINE PUSH-UP

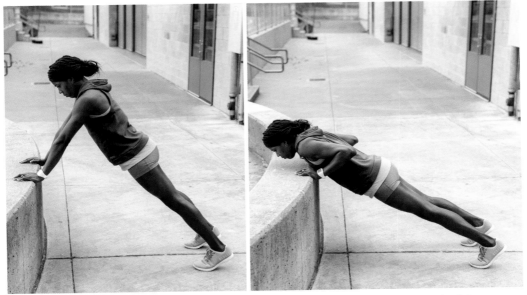

Get into push-up position, positioning your hands on a wall or high step. Keeping your body in a straight line, lower your body toward your hands, keeping your elbows tucked; then return to start. (If push-ups are hard for you, the incline will help build strength for a body-weight push-up.)

≫ INCLINE PUSH-UP, LEG EXTENDED

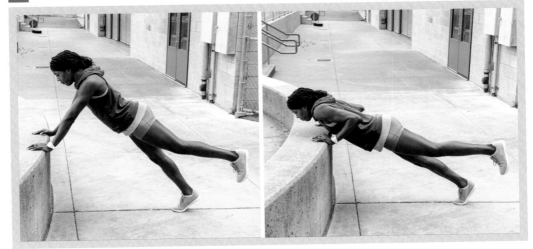

Now try it with one leg lifted. Work both sides.

2 | RAISE

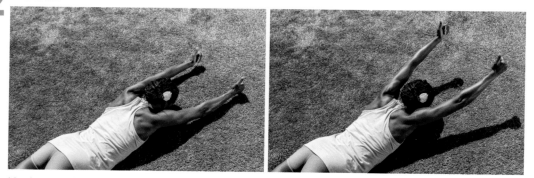

Lie down and squeeze your shoulder blades together to raise and lower your arms overhead in an "I" position, slow and controlled. Move from your shoulders, with your thumbs leading the way.

HIGH PLANK ▶ Hold 10–30 seconds for each set.

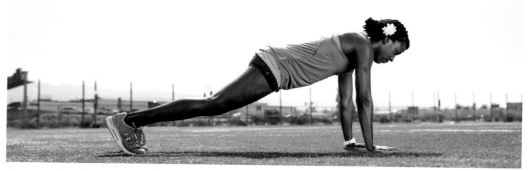

Place your hands under your shoulders and engage your core to hold your body in a straight line. ◀ To make this easier, drop to your knees.

≫ LOW PLANK ▶ Hold 10–30 seconds for each set.

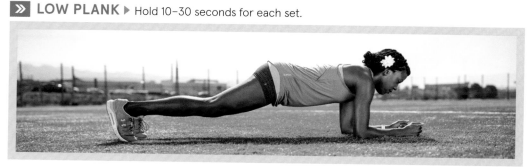

When you are ready for more, position your elbows under your shoulders, and engage your core, holding your body in a straight line. Fisted hands will help you get total-body tension for your low plank moves.

3 HIP THRUST

No bench?
Couches, sturdy chairs, and steps can all moonlight as a bench in a pinch!

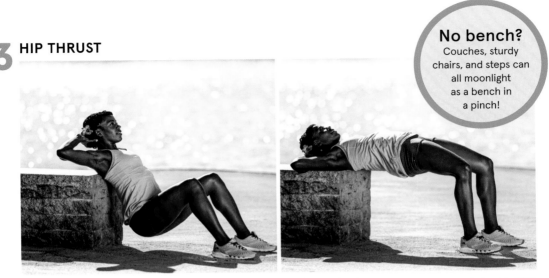

Place your shoulders on a bench and push down through your heels as you engage your glutes to raise your hips high. Pause at the top; then lower with control. Adjust your feet to be closer or farther away from your hips until you feel the work mostly in your glutes.

REVERSE PLANK ▶ Hold 10–20 seconds for each set.

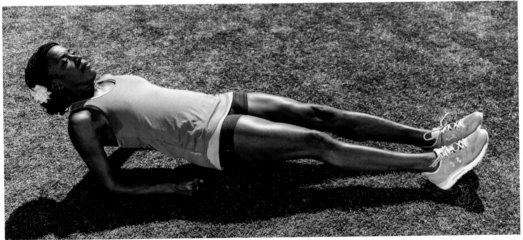

Lean back onto your elbows and engage your glutes, core, and back to hold your body in a straight line.

4 SIDE LUNGE

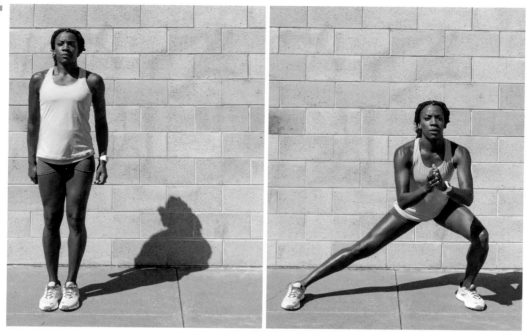

Step out to one side into a squat; then push off back to start. Work both sides.

Y RAISE

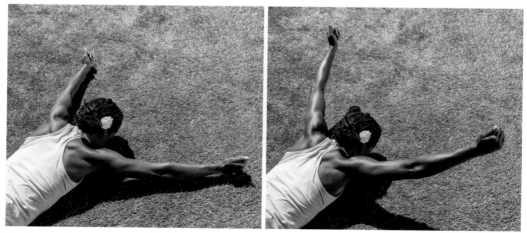

Lie down and squeeze your shoulder blades together to raise and lower your arms in a "Y" position, slow and controlled. Move from your shoulders, with your thumbs leading the way.

TEMPO RUN

Great for increasing your anaerobic threshold—helping you run harder, faster, without hitting the infamous wall—tempo runs are all about holding a nice, comfortable pace that you can maintain for long durations. The point here isn't to empty your tank. At the end of a tempo run, I want you to feel like you could keep going . . . if you wanted to.

WARM-UP

▶ Complete an easy 5-minute walk or jog to get your heart rate up and muscles ready to go. Aim for an average RPE of 3 to 4.

ACTIVATION DRILLS

▶ Do 6 reps of the following exercises, resting 15 seconds between each exercise.

FIRE HYDRANT

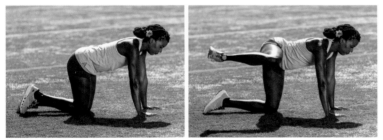

From an all-fours position, lift one leg out laterally, and lower it with control. Engage your core to keep your back flat and feel the glutes burn, even on the stationary leg. Work both sides.

DONKEY KICK

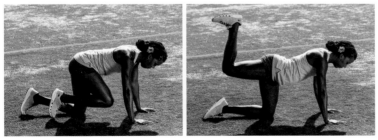

Now raise your foot up behind you and lower it back down with control. Work both sides.

INCHWORM

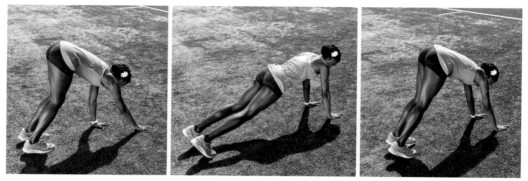

Get into a forward fold and walk your hands out into a high plank. Then walk your feet in until you are in a forward fold again. And keep on going.

HIGH-KNEE WALL HIKES

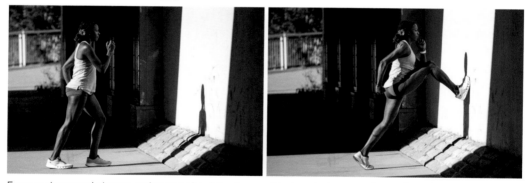

From a staggered stance, swing your back leg forward to touch down on the wall as close to hip-height as possible. Swing back to reload, pumping your arms in opposition with your legs. Work both sides.

RUN

TEMPO Run or jog for 20 minutes at tempo pace (RPE 6).

WEEKLY PROGRESSIONS

Your warm-up and tempo run will feel just as hard from week to week, but that's okay! You will likely be able to shave a few seconds off your pace from week to week as you get stronger, faster, and more confident!

CHALLENGE 1: KICK-START YOUR RUNNING RESOLUTION

▶ Hold each stretch
for 5 seconds, take a
breath, and see if you
can stretch a little farther.
Do this 5–6 times, then
repeat on the other side.

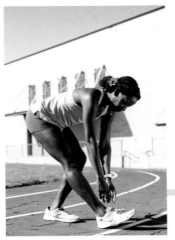

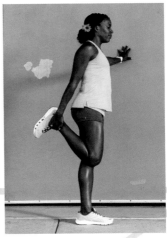

STANDING HAMSTRING STRETCH

Extend one leg just out in
front of you and let the knee
of the opposite leg bend
as you reach forward.
Try to keep your back flat.

STANDING QUAD STRETCH

Using a wall for support,
stand on one leg and pull the
opposite heel to your glute.
Press forward through your
stretched side to keep
your hips and knees square.

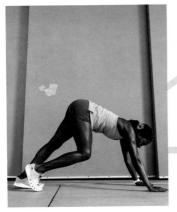

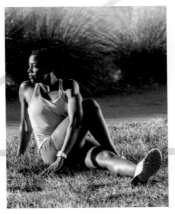

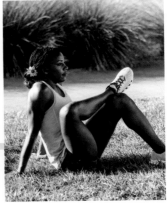

DOWNWARD DOG CALF STRETCH

Push your palms and heels
into the ground, bending one
knee at a time as you push
the opposite heel to the
ground to stretch that calf.

SEATED SPINAL ROTATION

With legs extended, cross one
leg over the other and twist
in the opposite direction,
using your arm to push your
knee in toward your chest.

SEATED GLUTE STRETCH

With knees bent, cross one
leg over the other to get into
a figure-4 position. Gently
move closer to your stationary
foot to intensify the stretch.

MOBILITY + LOW-INTENSITY STEADY STATE

Improve your range of motion while increasing core strength and stability—also vital to how you move—while giving extra love to often-cranky joints.

CIRCUIT 1

▶ Do 8 to 12 reps of exercises 1–5 back-to-back. Rest for 30 seconds; then repeat for a total of 3 rounds.

WEEKLY PROGRESSIONS

Week 2: Progress Superwoman to Twisting Superwoman
Week 3: Progress Mountain Climber to Twisting Mountain Climber
Week 4: Progress Hip Circles to Straight-Leg Hip Circles

1 SUPERWOMAN

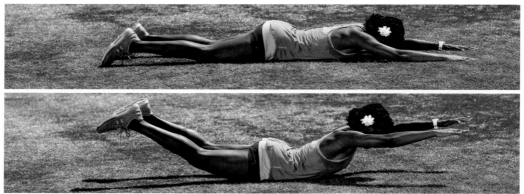

Extend your arms and engage your trunk muscles to lift your arms and legs; then lower back down with control. Back off the lift slightly if you feel the load in your low back.

≫ TWISTING SUPERWOMAN

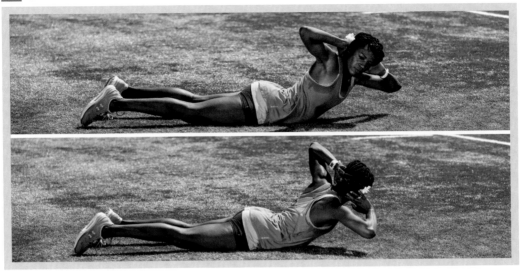

Lift and twist your torso from side to side with control.

2 HIP CIRCLES

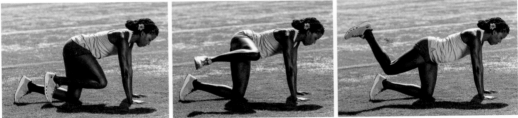

From an all-fours position, keep your core engaged as you lift your knee first out to the side, then around and behind you, and then forward to start another circle. Halfway through your reps, reverse direction. Work the other side.

≫ STRAIGHT-LEG HIP CIRCLES

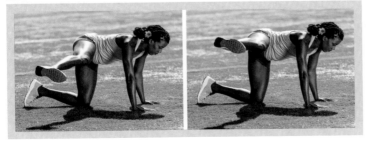

Engage your glutes to raise one leg straight out to your side. In one fluid motion, make a circle with your foot. Halfway through your reps, reverse direction. Work the other side.

3 T RAISE

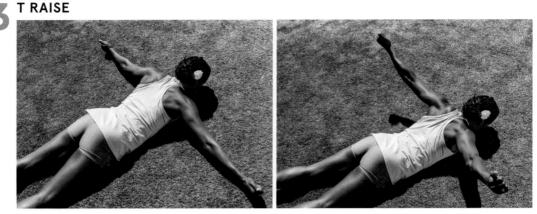

Lie down and squeeze your shoulder blades together to raise and lower your arms in a "T" position, slow and controlled. Move from your shoulders, with your thumbs leading the way.

4 MOUNTAIN CLIMBER

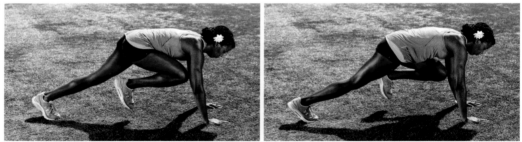

Get into a high-plank position and drive your knee in toward your chest—alternating sides. Get your feet moving, and keep your butt tucked. Engage your core and remember to breathe.

» TWISTING MOUNTAIN CLIMBER

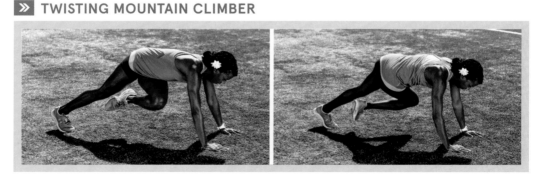

From high-plank position, bring your knee in toward the opposite elbow; alternate from side to side.

5 ALTERNATING HEEL SLIDE

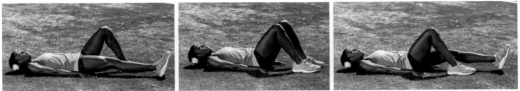

Lie down with your core engaged and your lower back flat on the ground. Slide your heel out and back in. Alternate sides.

▶ **Do 12 to 16 reps of exercises 6–9 back-to-back. Rest for 30 seconds; then repeat for a total of 2 rounds.**

6 BEAR CRAWL

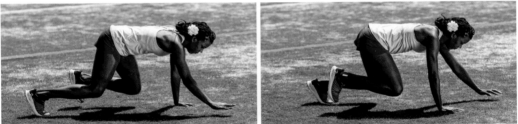

Come to your hands and the balls of your feet, and step forward with one hand and the opposite foot; then step with the opposing hand and foot. Keep your core engaged, back flat, and butt down. Halfway through the reps, move backward.

7 WALL SLIDE

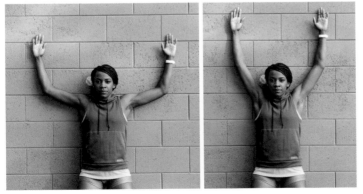

Stand with your butt, shoulders, elbows, and hands against the wall. Extend your arms up the wall, trying to limit the arch in your low back; then lower your body back down the wall. With practice, you'll be able to keep your low back closer to the wall and improve your range of motion.

8 HURDLE WALK-OVERS

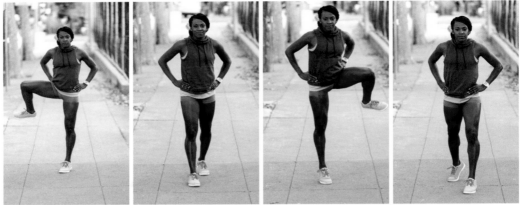

Lift one leg up and out to the side as if you were stepping over a hurdle and moving forward; continue alternating legs.

9 SIDE SHUFFLE

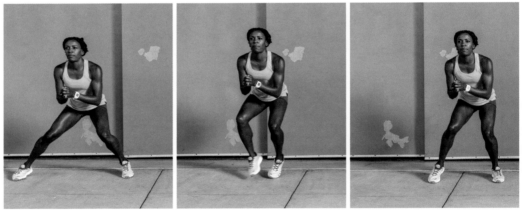

Squat slightly and shuffle with fast feet in one direction; then return the other direction.

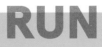

RUN

LOW-INTENSITY STEADY STATE Run or jog for 30 minutes at a pace that feels decidedly easy. Stick to an RPE of 4 to 5.

STRIDES

Kick your running into high gear with this stride workout. Performing strides will help you improve your running form and get a feel for speedwork.

WARM-UP

▶ Complete an easy 5-minute walk or jog to get your heart rate up and muscles ready to go. Aim for an average RPE of 3 to 4.

ACTIVATION DRILLS

▶ Do 6 reps of each exercise, resting 15 seconds between each set.

DONKEY KICK

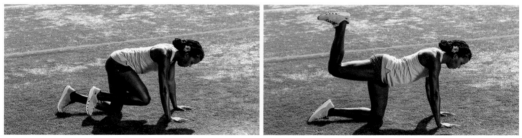

Get on all fours, and engage your glutes to raise your foot up behind you and lower it back down with control. Use your core to keep your back flat and feel the glutes burn, even on the stationary leg. Work both sides.

≫ DONKEY WHIP

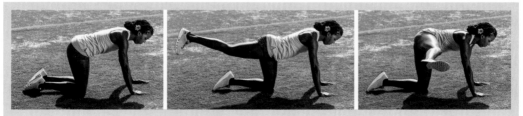

Extend one leg straight behind you; then whip it up to the side and back in a fluid, controlled motion. Engage your core and glute on the supporting side. Work both sides.

HIP THRUST

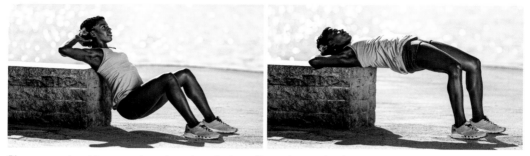

Place your shoulders on a bench and push down through your heels as you engage your glutes to raise your hips high. Pause at the top; then lower with control. Adjust your feet to be closer or farther away from your hips until you feel the work mostly in your glutes.

PLANK SHOULDER TAP

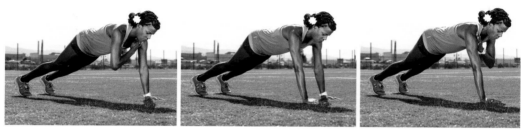

From high-plank position, stabilize yourself on one arm and tap your shoulder with the opposite hand. Alternate from side to side.

SINGLE-LEG DEADLIFT TO KNEE DRIVE

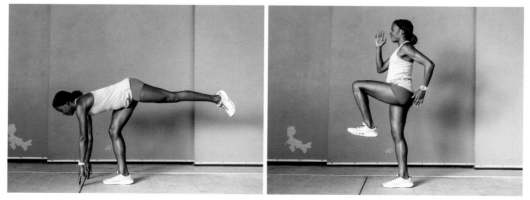

Balance on one leg, extending the opposite leg straight behind you, and tip forward. Keep your back flat and pendulum-swing your leg back up to a high-knee stance. Work both sides.

INCLINE PUSH-UP

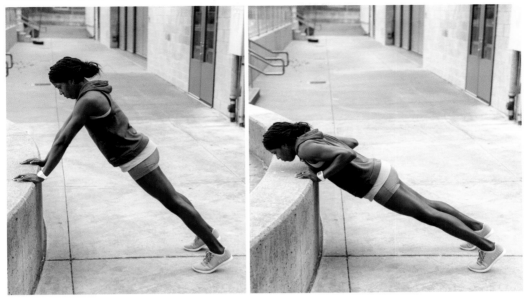

Get into push-up position, positioning your hands on a wall or high step. Keeping your body in a straight line, lower your body toward your hands, keeping your elbows tucked; then return to start.

RUN

STRIDES Do 4 sets of 20-second strides. Run at a comfortably hard pace (RPE 8), concentrating on an exaggerated, fluid form and big strides. Between sets, slow to a fast walk or slow jog until your heart rate comes down; then hit that next set stride.

WEEKLY PROGRESSION
Week 2: Increase to 5 sets of strides.
Week 3: Increase to 6 sets of strides.
Week 4: Increase to 7 sets of strides.

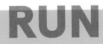

Fast, fluid, and controlled is the goal.

▶ Hold each stretch for 5 seconds, take a breath, and see if you can stretch a little farther. Do this 5–6 times, then repeat on the other side.

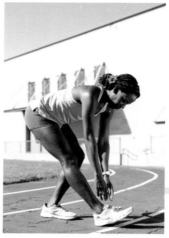

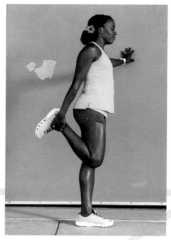

STANDING HAMSTRING STRETCH

Extend one leg just out in front of you and let the knee of the opposite leg bend as you reach forward. Try to keep your back flat.

STANDING QUAD STRETCH

Using a wall for support, stand on one leg and pull the opposite heel to your glute. Press forward through your stretched side to keep your hips and knees square.

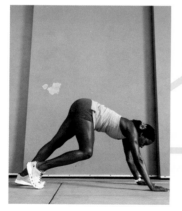

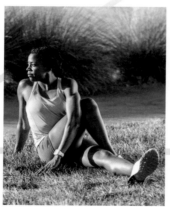

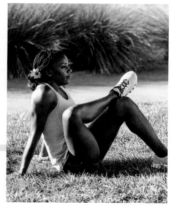

DOWNWARD DOG CALF STRETCH

Push your palms and heels into the ground, bending one knee at a time as you push the opposite heel to the ground to stretch that calf.

SEATED SPINAL ROTATION

With legs extended, cross one leg over the other and twist in the opposite direction, using your arm to push your knee in toward your chest.

SEATED GLUTE STRETCH

With knees bent, cross one leg over the other to get into a figure-4 position. Gently move closer to your stationary foot to intensify the stretch.

Challenge 2

MAKE-IT-FUN PARTNER SERIES

There's no community like the running community! It's home to some of the most inspiring and encouraging people I have ever met, and who understand the life-changing effects of movement. Running has taught them that there is no end to their power and potential to overcome challenges in every area of their lives.

My running community has supported me as a busy mother and runtrepreneur and, without these people, I would not be where I am today. I'm confident that you will find them equally supportive in your running journey.

This challenge celebrates the beauty of the running community and your place within it.

Each week, you'll perform five fun, 20- to 30-minute partner workouts that are designed to help you build running confidence. (Choose a partner who has a positive attitude and is truly invested.)

If you and your running buddy aren't able to meet up for every workout, that doesn't mean that you can't support each other in every workout! Call or text each other with words of encouragement. Set a time when you'll do the workout in your city, and they will do it in theirs. You can even have virtual partner sessions—days 2 and 4 are best for that.

Have fun with it and know that, wherever you are on your running journey, the running community is lucky to have you along!

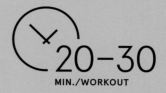

20–30
MIN./WORKOUT

5 days per week for *2 weeks*

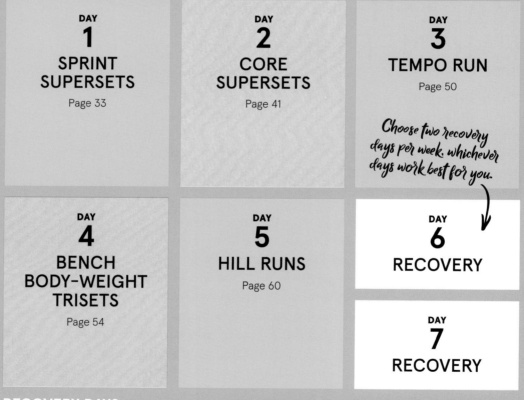

DAY **1** SPRINT SUPERSETS Page 33	DAY **2** CORE SUPERSETS Page 41	DAY **3** TEMPO RUN Page 50
DAY **4** BENCH BODY-WEIGHT TRISETS Page 54	DAY **5** HILL RUNS Page 60	DAY **6** RECOVERY
		DAY **7** RECOVERY

Choose two recovery days per week, whichever days work best for you.

RECOVERY DAYS If you do want to get a little recovery work in, check out the **Foam Rolling** and **Mobility** routines in the Appendix (p. 270).

EQUIPMENT Running shoes ▪ 2 resistance bands (1 short, 1 long) per partner ▪ foam roller

SPRINT SUPERSETS

This short-and-sweet workout will help you two pick up speed and strength!

WARM-UP

▶ Walk or jog for 5 minutes at a nice, easy pace that allows you two to chat (RPE 3 to 4).

ACTIVATION DRILLS

▶ Do 6 reps of each exercise in the superset, resting 15 seconds between each round. Do 3 rounds; then move on to the next superset. Work with your partner on these drills!

1 DEAD BUG

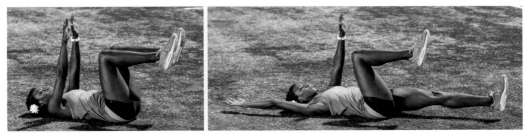

Get set with your low back flat on the ground, arms extended up, knees bent. Now move your opposing arm and leg to reach long while you move the opposite hand toward your knee. Keep alternating the movement, slow and controlled.

REVERSE PLANK ▶ Hold 10–20 seconds for each set.

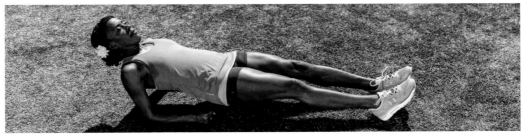

Lean back onto your elbows and engage your glutes, core, and back to hold your body in a straight line.

2 FORWARD LEG SWING

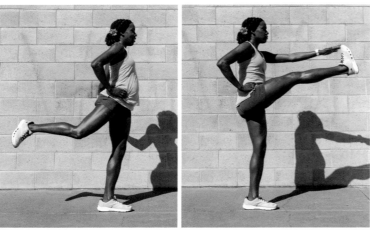

Swing one leg forward and back. Hold a wall for stability if needed. Repeat on the other side.

SIDEWAYS LEG SWING

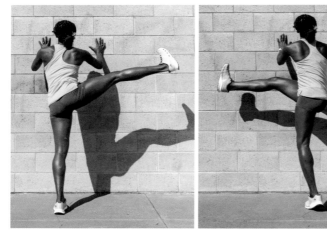

Face the wall and swing one leg from side to side. Work the other side.

FLOWER POWER

Community

Don't try to go it alone—whether in fitness or in life. Remember to look to your community as a source of inspiration and motivation when your own reserves are waning. It's a give-and-take thing because in the same way someone inspires you, you can inspire someone else to keep on going or strive for more. It's on all of us to ask for help and lift up our neighbor. And when we do it right, we leverage what makes each of us wonderfully unique and become stronger athletes and humans.

3 HIP CIRCLES

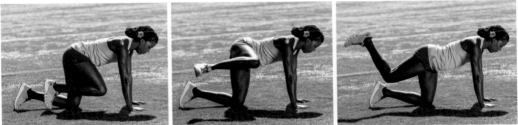

From an all-fours position, keep your core engaged as you lift your knee first out to the side, then around and behind you, and then forward to start another circle. Halfway through your reps, reverse direction. Work the other side.

MOUNTAIN CLIMBER

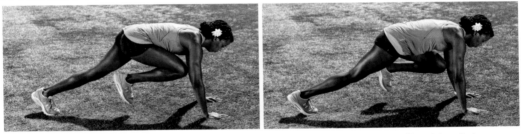

Get into a high-plank position and drive your knee in toward your chest—alternating sides. Get your feet moving, and keep your butt tucked.

4 ROLY-POLY POWER JUMP

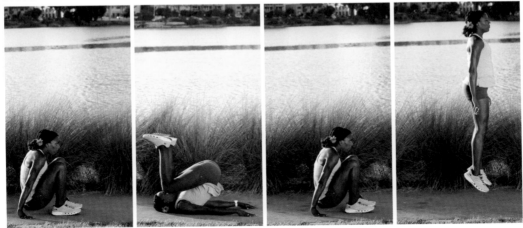

Start in a standing position, sit down, roll backward bringing your knees to chest; then quickly roll up onto your feet and power up into a jump.

JUMP ROPE

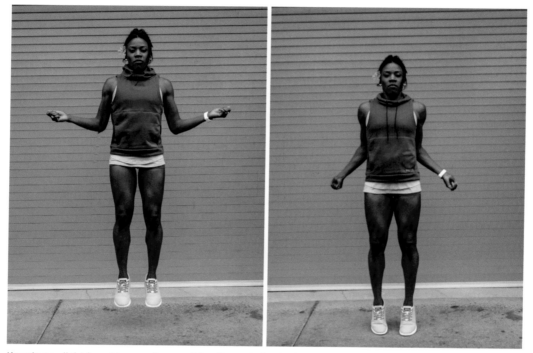

Keeping a slight bend in your knees, drive through the balls of your feet to bounce up and down as if you're jumping rope.

RUN

SPRINT + UPPER-BODY SUPERSETS Get started with a 30-second sprint (RPE 9), while your partner does the upper-body exercise for 30 seconds. Once you're finished, take a breather until you feel your heart rate come back down, and switch it up. Perform 1 go-around of each superset.

WEEKLY PROGRESSIONS
Your sprints will *always* feel hard, but see how far you can go in 30 seconds. I'm betting that you can add a few meters to your sprints from week to week! Also, if you're into it, during week 2, try performing 2 rounds of each superset. You've got this!

RUN

30-SECOND SPRINT

BAND PULL-APART

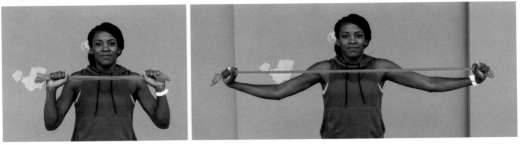

Hold the band palms out, with hands just outside of shoulder-width. Engage your core, squeeze your scapulas, and pull until your arms (and the band) are fully extended.

2

RUN

30-SECOND SPRINT

PLANK SHOULDER TAP

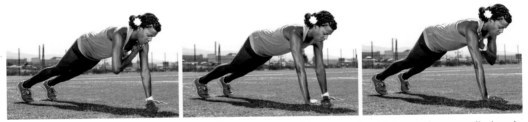

From high-plank position, stabilize yourself on one arm and tap your shoulder with the opposite hand. Alternate from side to side.

» WALK THE PLANK

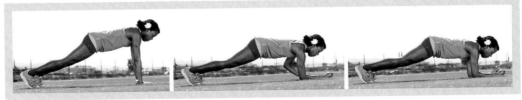

Move from a high plank to a low plank and back up again, keeping the movement going. Then switch it up to lead the up-down movement with the opposite arm. ◄ To make this easier, drop to your knees.

LAWNMOWER RESISTANCE BAND ROW

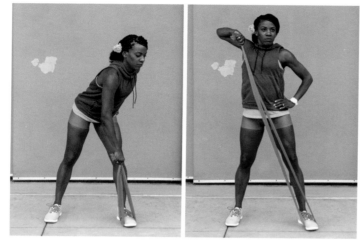

Anchor the band under one foot and hold it in the opposite hand. Pull the band up toward your shoulder, keeping your core engaged and elbow high. Return to the start position, slow and controlled. Work both sides.

BENT-OVER BAND ROW

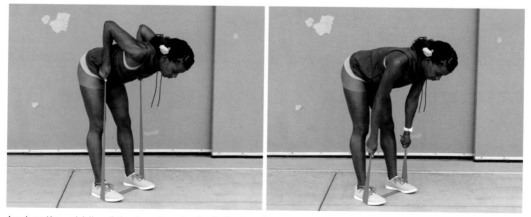

Anchor the middle of the band under both feet and hinge forward at the hips. Keeping your elbows tucked, pull the band up toward your chest. Return to the start position, slow and controlled.
▶ Wrap the band around your hands a few more times for greater resistance.

30-SECOND SPRINT

INCLINE PUSH-UP

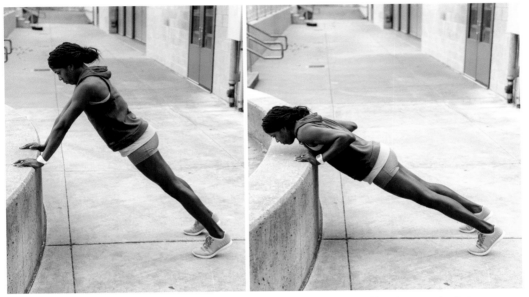

Get into push-up position, positioning your hands on a wall or high step. Keeping your body in a straight line, lower your body toward your hands, keeping your elbows tucked; then return to start.

≫ PUSH-UP

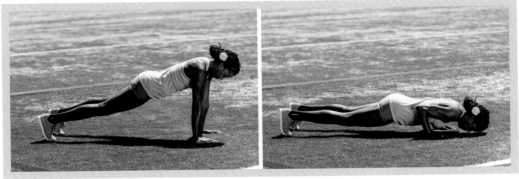

With your hands under your shoulders, squeeze your back, abs, and glutes to hold your body in a straight line. Lower your body to the ground, keeping your elbows tucked; then press back up.
≪ To make this easier, widen your feet.

▶ Hold each stretch for 5 seconds, take a breath, and see if you can stretch a little farther. Do this 5–6 times, then repeat on the other side.

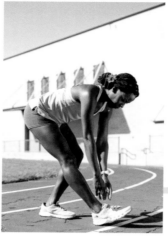

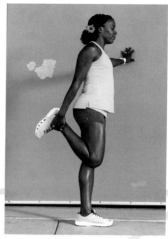

STANDING HAMSTRING STRETCH

Extend one leg just out in front of you and let the knee of the opposite leg bend as you reach forward. Try to keep your back flat.

STANDING QUAD STRETCH

Using a wall for support, stand on one leg and pull the opposite heel to your glute. Press forward through your stretched side to keep your hips and knees square.

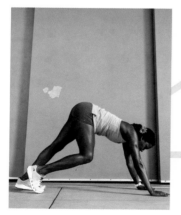

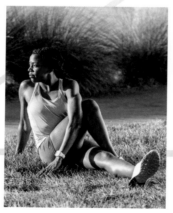

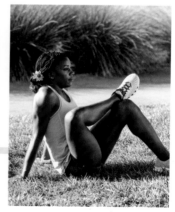

DOWNWARD DOG CALF STRETCH

Push your palms and heels into the ground, bending one knee at a time as you push the opposite heel to the ground to stretch that calf.

SEATED SPINAL ROTATION

With legs extended, cross one leg over the other and twist in the opposite direction, using your arm to push your knee in toward your chest.

SEATED GLUTE STRETCH

With knees bent, cross one leg over the other to get into a figure-4 position. Gently move closer to your stationary foot to intensify the stretch.

CORE SUPERSETS

The core is the center of everything you do in life: It doesn't matter if you're running, carrying around grocery bags or kiddos, dancing with friends, or sitting in a desk chair. Let's make your core strong and stable!

WARM-UP

▶ **Do 6 reps of exercises 1–4, back-to-back without rest. Do a total of 3 rounds, resting 15 seconds between each round. You and your partner can stay together!**

1 HIGH PLANK ▶ Hold 10–30 seconds for each set.

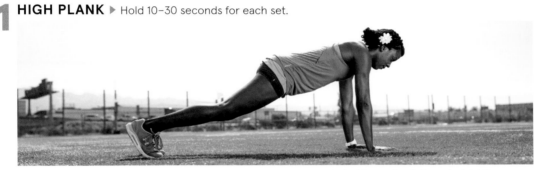

Place your hands under your shoulders and engage your core to hold your body in a straight line.
« To make this easier, drop to your knees.

2 HIP SWITCH

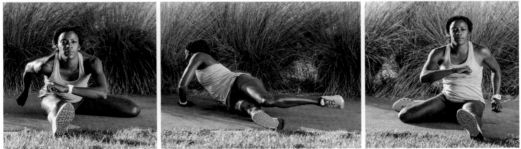

Sit with one leg extended and your other leg bent at a 90-degree angle behind you. Lean forward with the opposite arm leading the stretch. Now swing your back leg around and roll laterally into a stretch on the opposite side. Find your rhythm, moving dynamically from side to side.

3 BAND PULL-APART

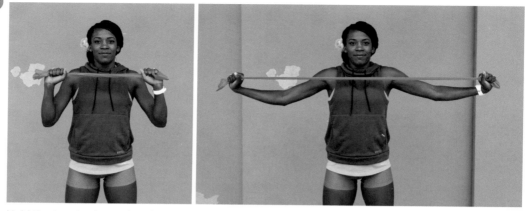

Hold the band palms out, with hands just outside of shoulder-width. Engage your core, squeeze your scapulas, and pull until your arms (and the band) are fully extended.

4 WALL SLIDE

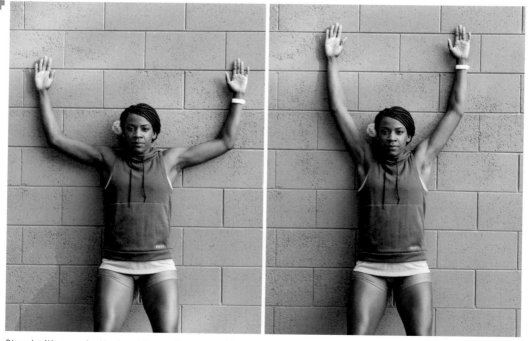

Stand with your butt, shoulders, elbows, and hands against the wall. Extend your arms up the wall, trying to limit the arch in your low back; then lower your body back down the wall. With practice, you'll be able to keep your low back closer to the wall and improve your range of motion.

▶ One of you will get started with the first exercise in the superset, and the other person will do the second exercise. Do your exercise for 30 seconds, take a short break, and then switch exercises. Perform 3 rounds of each superset.

WEEKLY PROGRESSIONS

With timed sets, track how many reps you can fit in. See if you can hold your rep count or add at least 1 extra rep within that 30-second window! Work in a new exercise progression when you feel ready. Don't sandbag!

1 BEAR CRAWL

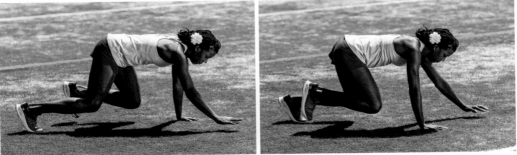

Come to your hands and the balls of your feet, and step forward with one hand and the opposite foot; then step with the opposing hand and foot. Keep your core engaged, back flat, and butt down. Halfway through the reps, move backward.

INCHWORM

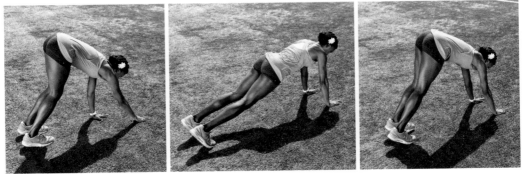

Get into a forward fold and walk your hands out into a high plank. Then walk your feet in until you are in a forward fold again. And keep on going.

2 CRUNCH TWIST

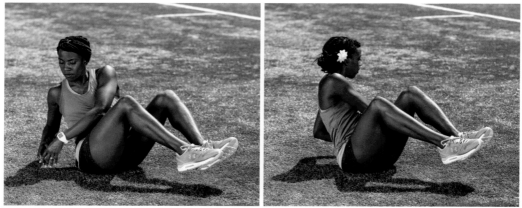

Engage your core and lift your feet off the ground, balancing on your butt. Rotate your torso as you twist from side to side, tracking your hands with your eyes.

ALTERNATING HEEL SLIDE

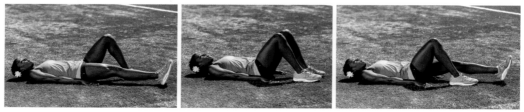

Lie down with your core engaged and your lower back flat on the ground. Slide your heel out and back in. Alternate sides.

» DOUBLE HEEL SLIDE

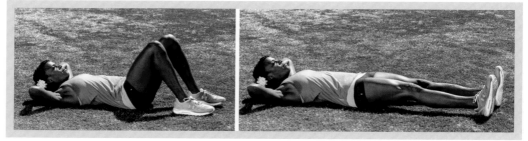

Slide both heels out and back in, keeping your core engaged and your low back flat.

3 LYING SCISSOR KICK

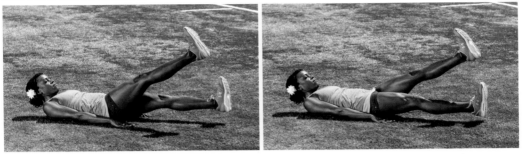

Engage your core, holding your shoulders and legs just off the ground as you "scissor" your legs up, then back down. Keep your low back flat on the ground.

CRUNCH

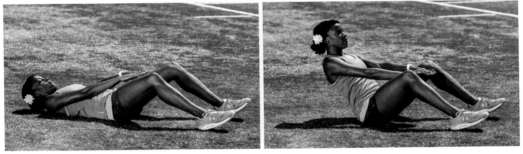

Engage your abs to lift your shoulders up and reach forward toward your knees; then come back down with control. Keep going. Note that this is not a full sit-up. Crunch until your abdominal wall starts to feel angry; then lower back down and keep it going.

» SPLIT-LEG CRUNCH

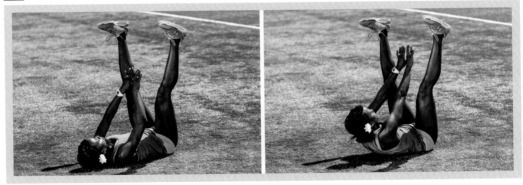

With legs extended, engage your abs to raise your shoulders and reach; then come back down with control. Keep your back flat and legs still.

4 SIDE PLANK ▶ Hold 10–20 seconds for each set.

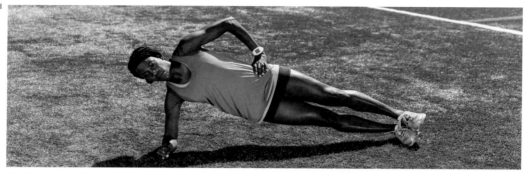

Position your elbow under your shoulder and lift your hips until your body is in a straight line. Work the other side.

» SIDE PLANK WITH HIP DIP

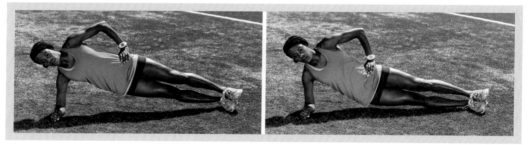

From a side plank, drop your hips down toward the ground and raise them back up into alignment. Work both sides.

SPLIT-LEG CROSS-TOE TOUCH

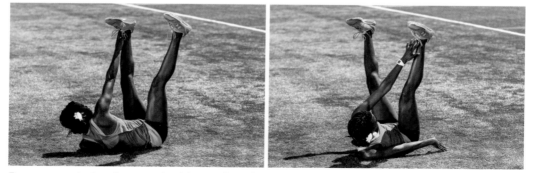

Engage your abs to raise your shoulders and reach your hand to the opposite foot; then come back down with control. Alternate sides, keeping your back flat and legs still.

≫ LYING CROSS-TOE TOUCH

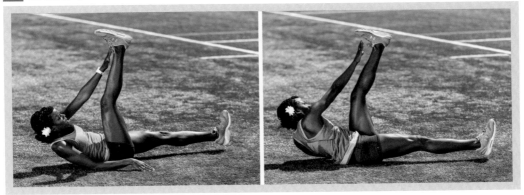

Lie down and engage your abs as you lift your heels off the ground. Reach one hand for the opposite foot as you lift your leg. Alternate sides, keeping your lower back flat and arms and legs straight.

5 COBRA SUPERWOMAN

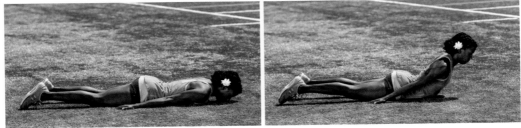

Start with your arms at your sides, palms down, and engage your trunk muscles to lift and lower your torso with control. Back off the lift slightly if you feel the load in your low back.

≫ SUPERWOMAN

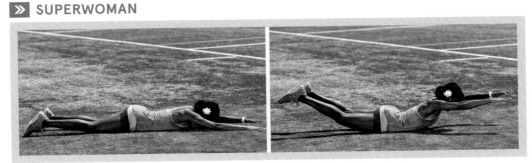

Extend your arms and engage your trunk muscles to lift your arms and legs; then lower back down with control. Back off the lift slightly if you feel the load in your low back.

LOW PLANK ▶ Hold 10–30 seconds for each set.

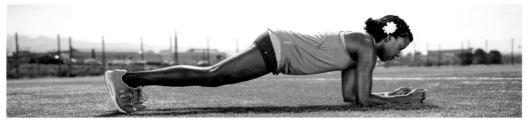

Position your elbows under your shoulders, and engage your core, holding your body in a straight line.
« To make this easier, drop to your knees.

≫ LOW PLANK WITH LEG LIFT

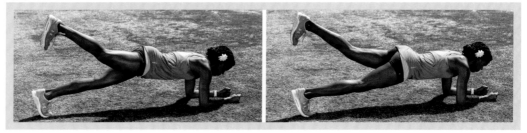

From a low plank position, engage your core and lift one leg, then the other. Keep your hips steady as you continue the leg lifts.

COOLDOWN

▶ We're sandwiching today's workout with the same warm-up and cooldown.
Do 6 reps of exercises 1–4 back-to-back without rest. Take a short breather; then repeat for a total of 3 rounds. You and your partner can stay together!

1 HIGH PLANK ▶ Hold 10–30 seconds for each set.

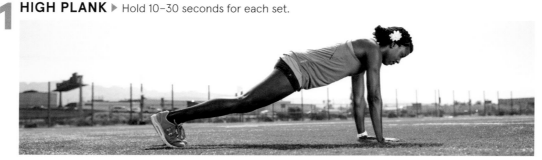

Place your hands under your shoulders and engage your core to hold your body in a straight line.
« To make this easier, drop to your knees.

2 HIP SWITCH

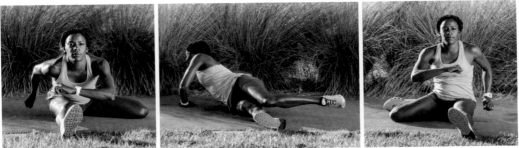

Sit with one leg extended and your other leg bent at a 90-degree angle behind you. Lean forward with the opposite arm leading the stretch. Now swing your back leg around and roll laterally into a stretch on the opposite side. Find your rhythm, moving dynamically from side to side.

3 BAND PULL-APART

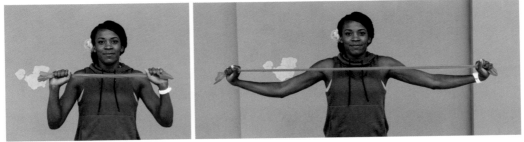

Hold the band palms out, with hands just outside of shoulder-width. Engage your core, squeeze your scapulas, and pull until your arms (and the band) are fully extended.

4 WALL SLIDE

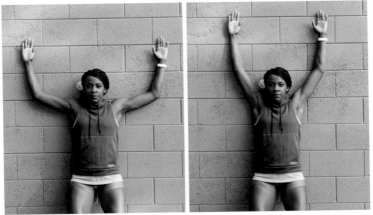

Stand with your butt, shoulders, elbows, and hands against the wall. Extend your arms up the wall, trying to limit the arch in your low back; then lower your body back down the wall.

TEMPO RUN

Great for boosting your anaerobic threshold (that point when you can no longer talk easily), tempo runs will help you run faster and longer. They involve holding a nice, comfortable pace that you can maintain for long durations. If you add about 1–2 minutes to your mile time trial pace, your ideal tempo pace is likely closer to 1 minute—work toward that goal. (We ran a 1-mile time trial in Challenge 1. Repeat this benchmark test at any time to help you plan your paces.)

WARM-UP

▶ Walk or jog for 5 minutes at a nice, easy pace that allows you two to chat.

ACTIVATION DRILLS

▶ Do 8 reps of each exercise, resting 15 seconds between exercise. You and your partner can stay together here!

BAND WALK

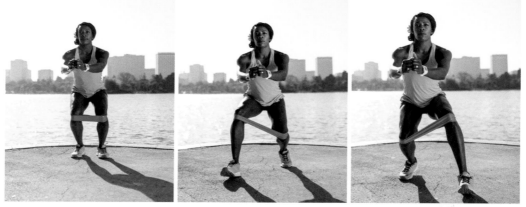

Place a band at or just above your knees. Start from a half-squat stance with your feet shoulder-width apart and walk forward, heel-to-toe, keeping the band taut. Halfway through the reps walk backward, toe-to-heel.

LATERAL BAND WALK

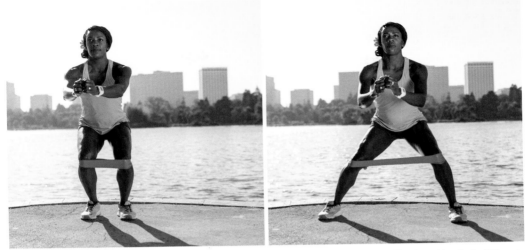

Now step one foot out to the side and follow with the opposite foot, keeping the band taut at all times. Return in the opposite direction to work the other side.

JACK SQUAT

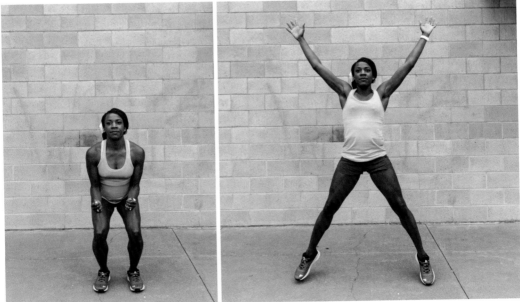

You don't know jack squat . . . yet! Start from a squat, arms tucked; then pop up and out into the jack position, legs and arms out. Spring from squat to jack and back without pausing.

RUNNING JACK

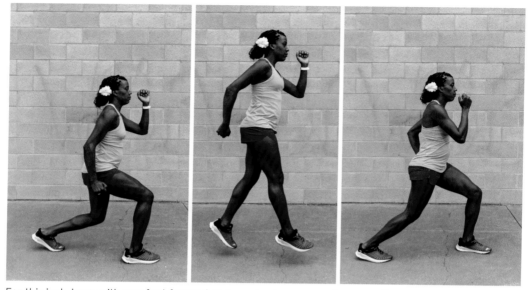

For this jack, jump with one foot forward and one back, arms moving opposite your legs.

RUN

TEMPO RUN   Run or jog for 20 minutes, focusing on keeping a challenging, but comfortable, pace that you feel you could keep going for 10 extra minutes (RPE 5 to 6). We're not trying to wipe each other out here, just get in some solid cardio and practice pacing.

WEEKLY PROGRESSIONS
See if you can shave a few seconds off your pace each week as you become stronger and more confident!

Shuttle it!
You and your workout buddy might have different tempo paces. That's okay! Here's a fun way to run together even if you're running at different speeds:

Set your watches or phones to beep every minute, and then get going! Every time your gadget beeps, turn around and start running in the opposite direction. By shuttling back and forth this way, you will always be running together! Sometimes you'll lead; sometimes your partner will; have fun with it!

▶ Hold each stretch for 5 seconds, take a breath, and see if you can stretch a little farther. Do this 5–6 times, then repeat on the other side.

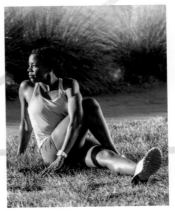

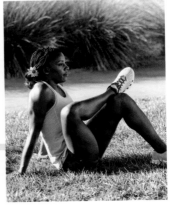

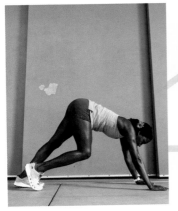

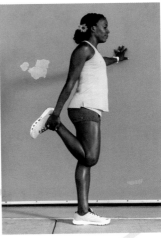

STANDING HAMSTRING STRETCH

Extend one leg just out in front of you and let the knee of the opposite leg bend as you reach forward. Try to keep your back flat.

STANDING QUAD STRETCH

Using a wall for support, stand on one leg and pull the opposite heel to your glute. Press forward through your stretched side to keep your hips and knees square.

DOWNWARD DOG CALF STRETCH

Push your palms and heels into the ground, bending one knee at a time as you push the opposite heel to the ground to stretch that calf.

SEATED SPINAL ROTATION

With legs extended, cross one leg over the other and twist in the opposite direction, using your arm to push your knee in toward your chest.

SEATED GLUTE STRETCH

With knees bent, cross one leg over the other to get into a figure-4 position. Gently move closer to your stationary foot to intensify the stretch.

BENCH BODY-WEIGHT TRISETS

Benches are awesome find-anywhere tools to challenge your body in new ways—and without having to lug around a set of weights.

WARM-UP

▶ Do 6 reps of each exercise in the superset, resting 15 seconds between each round. Do 3 rounds, then start the next superset. You and your partner can work together!

1 HIGH KNEES

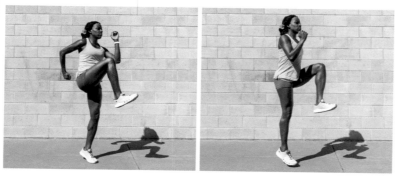

Drive one knee up, and feel the lift as you hop-skip up to the ball of your foot; alternate sides. Drive your arms in a tight stride, opposite your legs. This is a quick, stationary movement.

A-SKIP

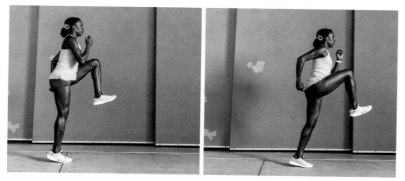

Hop-skip with high knees, swinging your arms to keep momentum.

2 LATERAL LADDER

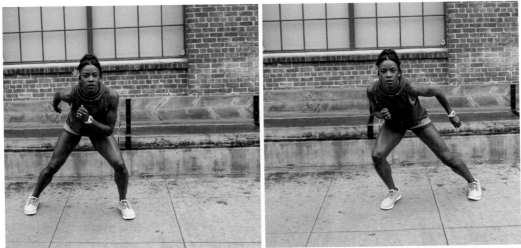

Get in a wide athletic stance and shuffle your feet from side to side, keeping your weight over the inside foot. Pump your arms for momentum and move as quickly as possible. Fast feet!

B-SKIP

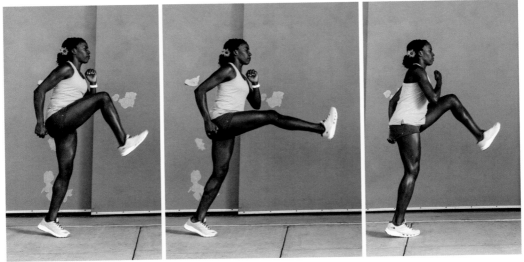

Hop-skip, engaging your glute to pull your knee up, then swing your leg forward to extension. Move your arms for momentum.

▶ Let's have some bench fun with trisets! These are groupings of three exercises that you perform back-to-back without rest. To do them, each of you will get started with a different exercise, perform it for 30 seconds, and then move onto the next in a mini-circuit. At the end of a round, get some water and let your heart rates come down to the point that you have the breath to talk each other up for the next go-around. Repeat for a total of 3 rounds; then do the next triset.

At the end of all trisets, follow up with the finisher—one last exercise to empty the tank. Perform as many reps as you can in a row!

1 BOX JUMP

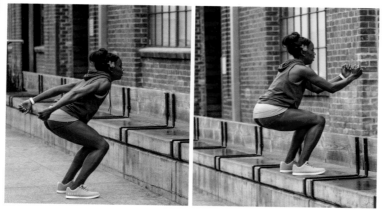

Swing your arms behind you as you squat down; then drive through your legs to explode up and forward. Land soft and come to a stand. Keep your hips tucked and step back down.

INCLINE PUSH-UP, LEG EXTENDED

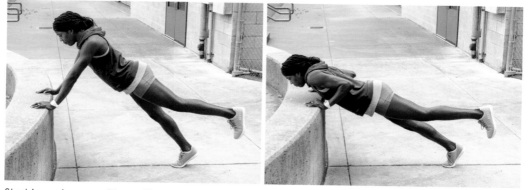

Start in push-up position, with one leg lifted, positioning your hands on a wall or high step. Keeping your body in a straight line, lower your body toward your hands, keeping your elbows tucked; then return to start. Work both sides.

REAR-FOOT-ELEVATED SPLIT SQUAT

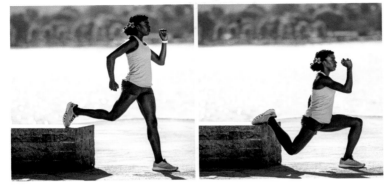

Stand on one leg and position your opposite foot behind you on a bench. Lower your hips down into a squat and drive through your heel to come back up. Work both sides.

2 STEP-UP

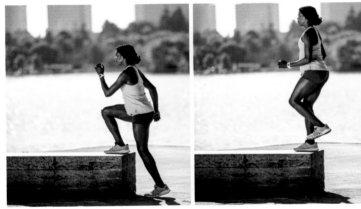

Start with one foot up on a bench or step. Drive through that leg as you explode up and raise your opposite knee toward your chest; then land soft and step back down. Keep a steady rhythm, moving your arms opposite your legs to create momentum. Work both sides.

» SINGLE-LEG POWER-UP

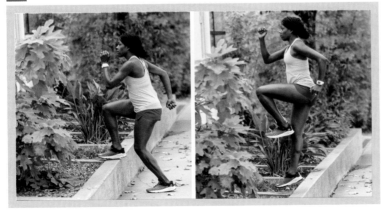

Start with one foot up on a bench or step. Drive through that leg as you explode up and raise your opposite knee toward your chest; then land soft and step back down. Keep a steady rhythm, moving your arms opposite your legs to create momentum. Work both sides.

INCLINE PUSH-UP

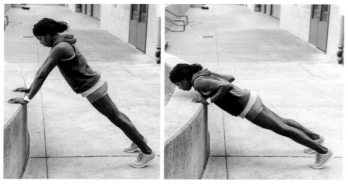

Get into push-up position, positioning your hands on a wall or high step. Keeping your body in a straight line, lower your body toward your hands, keeping your elbows tucked; then return to start.

HIP THRUST

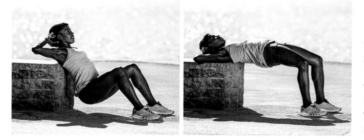

Place your shoulders on a bench and push down through your heels as you engage your glutes to raise your hips high. Pause at the top; then lower with control. Adjust your feet to be closer or farther away from your hips until you feel the work mostly in your glutes.

FINISHER

▶ **Perform as many reps of this exercise as you can to empty your tank.**

SINGLE-LEG SQUAT

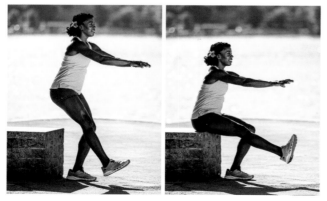

Stand on one leg and sit back until your butt lightly touches the bench. Press through the standing leg to return to standing. Extend your arms in front for balance as you squat down, slow and controlled. Work both sides.

▶ Hold each stretch
for 5 seconds, take a
breath, and see if you
can stretch a little farther.
Do this 5–6 times, then
repeat on the other side.

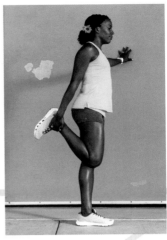

STANDING HAMSTRING STRETCH

Extend one leg just out in
front of you and let the knee
of the opposite leg bend
as you reach forward.
Try to keep your back flat.

STANDING QUAD STRETCH

Using a wall for support,
stand on one leg and pull the
opposite heel to your glute.
Press forward through your
stretched side to keep
your hips and knees square.

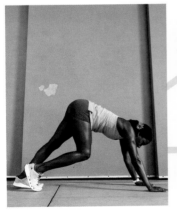

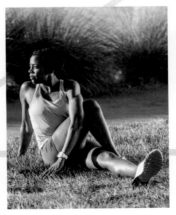

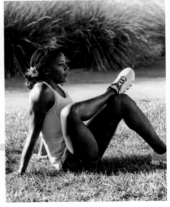

DOWNWARD DOG CALF STRETCH

Push your palms and heels
into the ground, bending one
knee at a time as you push
the opposite heel to the
ground to stretch that calf.

SEATED SPINAL ROTATION

With legs extended, cross one
leg over the other and twist
in the opposite direction,
using your arm to push your
knee in toward your chest.

SEATED GLUTE STRETCH

With knees bent, cross one
leg over the other to get into
a figure-4 position. Gently
move closer to your stationary
foot to intensify the stretch.

HILL RUNS

Despite what you might have heard, hills can be super fun! Go in knowing that it's supposed to be hard and that pushing through will work wonders for your speed and ability to accelerate quickly—whether it be at the beginning of a race, on a challenging course, when a competitor puts in a surge for you to match, or when it's time to put down the hammer. Hills are for breakfast, lunch, and dinner!

WARM-UP

▶ Walk or jog for 5 minutes at a nice, easy pace that allows you two to chat.

ACTIVATION DRILLS

▶ Do 6 reps of each exercise in the superset, resting 15 seconds between each round. Do 3 rounds, then the next superset. You and your partner can stay together here!

1 SKATER JUMP

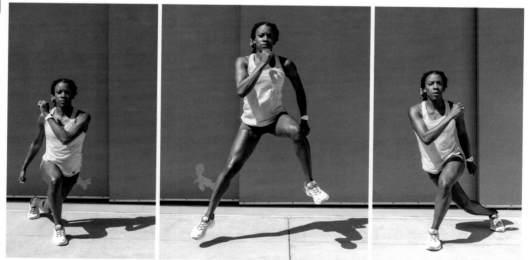

Jump from side to side. As you land, swing the inside leg behind you and touch down lightly before bounding back to the other side.

SINGLE-LEG DEADLIFT TO KNEE DRIVE

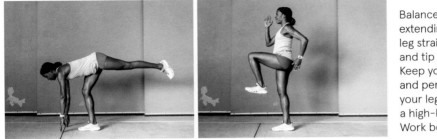

Balance on one leg, extending the opposite leg straight behind you, and tip forward. Keep your back flat and pendulum-swing your leg back up to a high-knee stance. Work both sides.

2 HURDLE WALK-OVERS

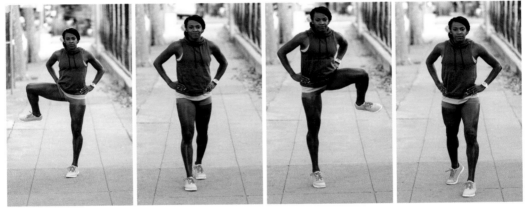

Lift one leg up and out to the side as if you were stepping over a hurdle and moving forward; continue alternating legs.

SIDE HURDLE

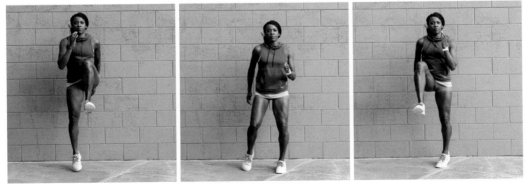

Lift one leg up and step out to the side as if you are stepping over a hurdle, and follow with the trailing leg coming up and over the hurdle. Keep it going, and halfway through the reps, switch direction.

3 LATERAL BAND WALK

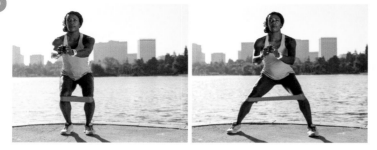

Place the band just below your knees. From a half-squat stance, step one foot out to the side and follow with the opposite foot, keeping the band taut at all times. Return in the opposite direction to work the other side.

BAND WALK

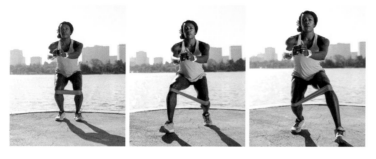

Stand with your feet shoulder-width apart and walk forward, heel-to-toe, keeping the band taut. Halfway through the reps walk backward, toe-to-heel.

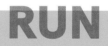

HILLS Pick a hill and run up it as fast as you can (RPE 7 to 8)! It doesn't have to be long—make it a 20- or 30-second sprint. Once you reach the top, take a few deep breaths and slowly walk down the hill to let your heart rate come back down to normal. Repeat. You two can take turns running or run together. Depending on the length and height of the hill, aim for anywhere from 5 to 10 hill runs.

Finding hills near you

Depending on where you live, hills may be in short supply. Building entrance ramps and parking garages (watch for cars!) can be super-convenient "hills." In a pinch, you can also run up the stairs in your house, apartment building, or office. If you have a treadmill or gym membership, set the treadmill incline at a level that allows you to run *without* holding onto the handrails!

WEEKLY PROGRESSIONS
How many hill runs did you get in during week 1? Add 1 more with each week in the challenge or step up your interval time by 10 seconds with each week.

▶ Hold each stretch for 5 seconds, take a breath, and see if you can stretch a little farther. Do this 5–6 times, then repeat on the other side.

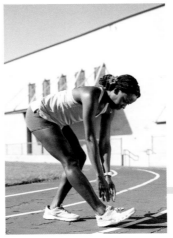

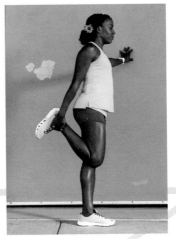

STANDING HAMSTRING STRETCH

Extend one leg just out in front of you and let the knee of the opposite leg bend as you reach forward. Try to keep your back flat.

STANDING QUAD STRETCH

Using a wall for support, stand on one leg and pull the opposite heel to your glute. Press forward through your stretched side to keep your hips and knees square.

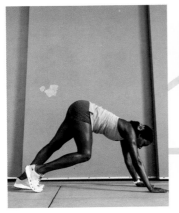

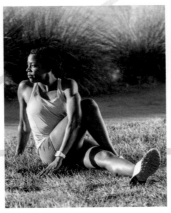

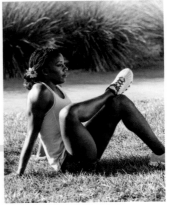

DOWNWARD DOG CALF STRETCH

Push your palms and heels into the ground, bending one knee at a time as you push the opposite heel to the ground to stretch that calf.

SEATED SPINAL ROTATION

With legs extended, cross one leg over the other and twist in the opposite direction, using your arm to push your knee in toward your chest.

SEATED GLUTE STRETCH

With knees bent, cross one leg over the other to get into a figure-4 position. Gently move closer to your stationary foot to intensify the stretch.

Challenge 3

FIT IN FITNESS

This challenge is for the realest of humans. The ones who hustle, juggle, and far too often put themselves at the bottom of their to-do list. Let's face it: That's most of us.

This seven-day challenge will help you reboot when it feels like life is on the fritz. When you feel that all the *-nesses* (busyness, messiness, overwhelming-ness) of life are eating up your running routine. You might be thinking, *Seven days?!? There's no way I can work out every day of the week!*

I'm here to tell you that with the right strategy, you totally can! Comprised of 15-minute workouts—and 5-minute supersets or "mini-workouts" within them—this challenge teaches you how to integrate movement into real life. No 30-minute-plus workout windows or elaborate equipment required.

Whether you're at home, on the road, or all around town in a frenzy of to-dos, just a few minutes here and there throughout the day add up. They add up to a fitter, healthier, happier you.

Affirmation

Take time to write down your truths. These are reminders of all the great things you know to be true about yourself, things you have accomplished and overcome. These truths can get lost in the big sea of obstacles and struggles. Post them as reminders of the best version of you. We all need to be reminded of what we are made of and what makes us great.

FLOWER POWER

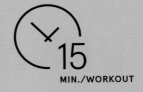

15 MIN./WORKOUT

Each workout can be broken into 3 mini-workouts.

7 days *(1 week)*

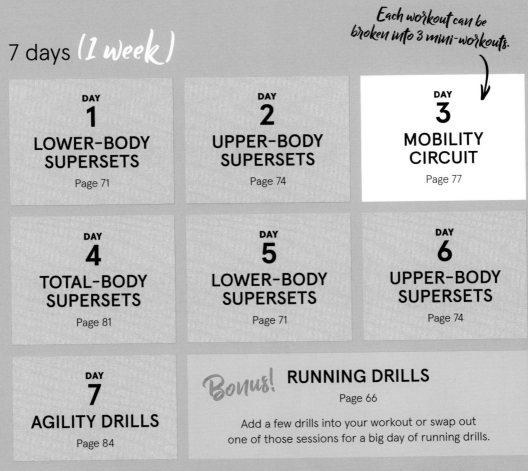

DAY 1
LOWER-BODY SUPERSETS
Page 71

DAY 2
UPPER-BODY SUPERSETS
Page 74

DAY 3
MOBILITY CIRCUIT
Page 77

DAY 4
TOTAL-BODY SUPERSETS
Page 81

DAY 5
LOWER-BODY SUPERSETS
Page 71

DAY 6
UPPER-BODY SUPERSETS
Page 74

DAY 7
AGILITY DRILLS
Page 84

Bonus! **RUNNING DRILLS**
Page 66

Add a few drills into your workout or swap out one of those sessions for a big day of running drills.

EQUIPMENT Running shoes ▪ 2 resistance bands (1 short, 1 long) ▪ dumbbells ▪ box or step

Think outside the box

Don't limit your fitness to formal workouts! Everyday to-dos like mowing the yard, washing the car, cleaning the baseboards, and carrying groceries will help you work up a sweat. So do a few shoulder presses with a gallon of milk and give yourself the credit you deserve!

Bonus!
RUNNING DRILLS

On the days when you don't have time for a run you can fit in a few of these running drills—just enough agility and quickness to make you feel great. Here are my favorites:

Do 12–16 reps or 30-second intervals. Fit in sets as time allows.

HIGH KNEES

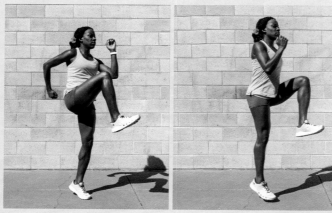

Drive one knee up, and feel the lift as you hop-skip up to the ball of your foot; alternate sides. Drive your arms in a tight stride, opposite your legs.

SPLIT SQUAT JUMP

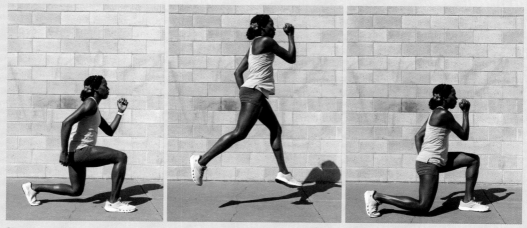

Start in a split stance and pop up. Switch your stance as you hit the height of your jump and land soft. Get your arms moving opposite your legs so you can tap that momentum.

SKATER JUMP

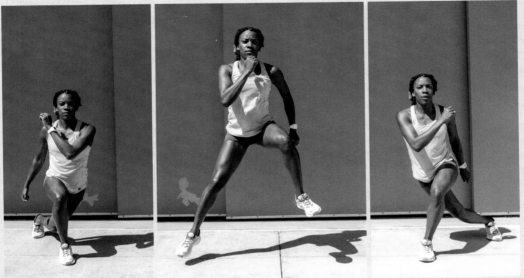

Jump from side to side. As you land, swing the inside leg behind you and touch down lightly before bounding back to the other side.

SINGLE-LEG DEADLIFT TO KNEE DRIVE

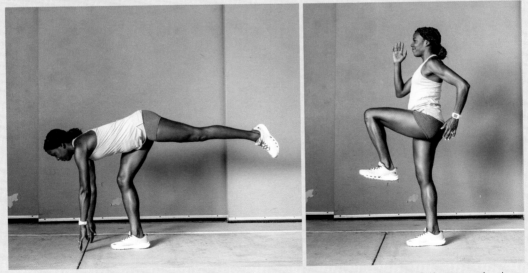

Balance on one leg, extending the opposite leg straight behind you and tip forward. Keep your back flat and pendulum-swing your leg back up to a high-knee stance. Work both sides.

SIDE SHUFFLE

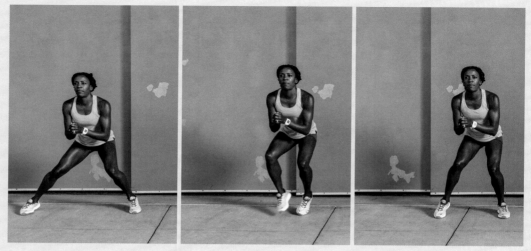

Squat slightly and shuffle with fast feet in one direction; then return the other direction.

A-SKIP

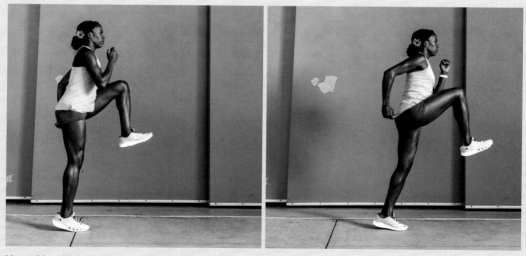

Hop-skip with high knees, swinging your arms to keep momentum.

CHALLENGE 3: FIT IN FITNESS

B-SKIP

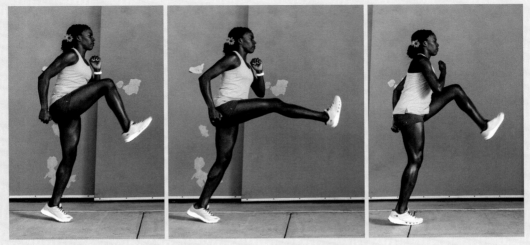

Hop-skip, engaging your glute to pull your knee up (like the A-Skip), then swing your leg forward to extension. Move your arms for momentum.

JUMP ROPE

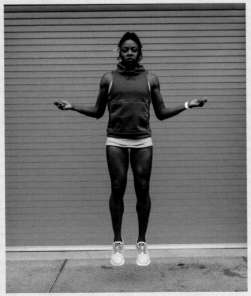

Keeping a slight bend in your knees, drive through the balls of your feet to bounce up and down as if you're jumping rope.

» SINGLE-LEG JUMP ROPE

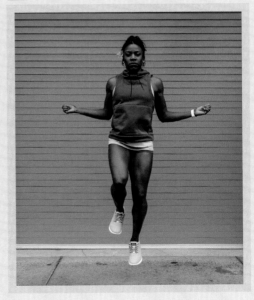

Stand on one leg and keep a slight bend in your knee, and drive through the ball of your foot to bounce up and down as if you're jumping rope. Switch legs.

X JUMP

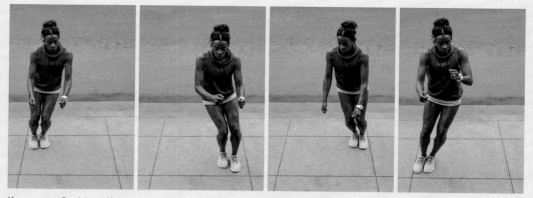

Keep your feet together as you jump from corner to corner, hitting all four corners of a square—diagonally forward, back, diagonally forward, then back to the first corner. Switch directions halfway through the rep count.

LATERAL LADDER

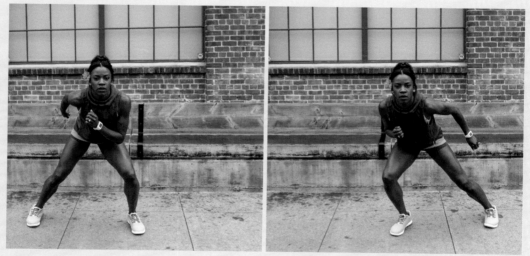

Get in a wide athletic stance and shuffle your feet from side to side, keeping your weight over the inside foot. Pump your arms for momentum and move as quickly as possible. Fast feet!

LOWER-BODY SUPERSETS

Strengthen your glutes, hamstrings, and quads with powerful multi-joint moves. Here, you'll alternate between exercises that focus on your backside, or posterior chain, and the front of your legs, also known as your anterior chain.

▶ Perform the supersets by completing 8 to 12 reps of both exercises in the set. Rest for 30 seconds; then repeat the superset for a total of 3 to 4 rounds. Make sure to check off each superset by the end of the day.

1 BAND WALK

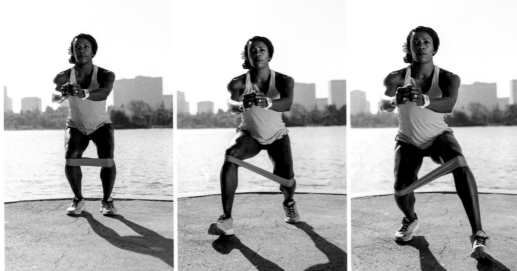

Place the band at or just above your knees. Start from a half-squat stance with your feet shoulder-width apart and walk forward, heel-to-toe, keeping the band taut. Halfway through the reps walk backward, toe-to-heel.

WALKING LUNGE

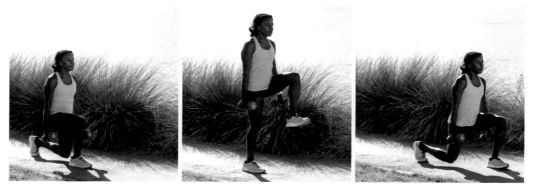

Step into a lunge, sinking down until your quad is parallel with the ground. Push off your back foot and bring your knee high before stepping forward into a lunge on the opposite side. Let your legs do the work.

 ## SIDE LUNGE TO KNEE DRIVE

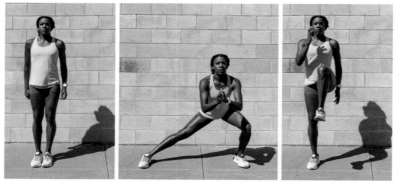

Step out to one side into a squat; then push up into a sprinter position, knee high. Work both sides.

REAR-FOOT-ELEVATED SPLIT SQUAT

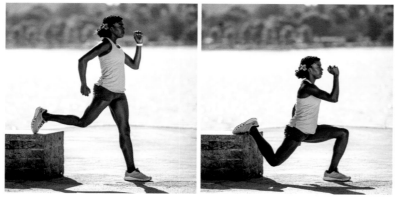

Stand on one leg and position your opposite foot behind you on a bench. Lower your hips down into a squat and drive through your heel to come back up. Work both sides.

3 HIGH KNEES

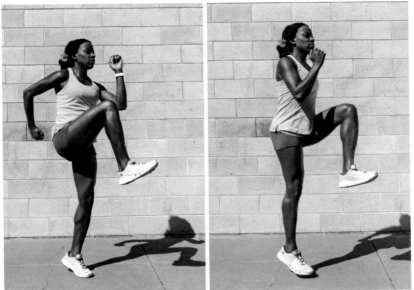

Drive one knee up, and feel the lift as you hop-skip up to the ball of your foot; alternate sides. Drive your arms in a tight stride, opposite your legs.

SINGLE-LEG SQUAT

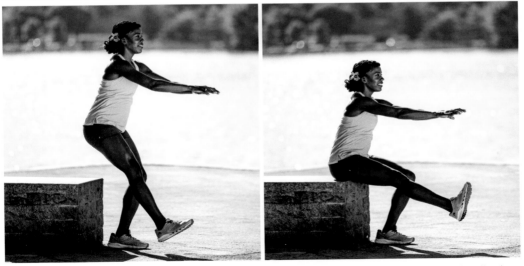

Stand on one leg and sit back until your butt lightly touches the bench. Press through the standing leg to return to standing. Extend your arms in front for balance as you squat down, slow and controlled. Work both sides. ▶▶ When you feel confident, you can ditch the bench and make this an unassisted pistol squat. (I'm an Olympic athlete, and I still opt for a bench!)

UPPER-BODY SUPERSETS

Upper-body work requires either pulling or pushing. By alternating back and forth between pushing and pulling exercises, you'll strengthen your arms, chest, and back in record time.

▶ Do the supersets by performing 8 to 12 reps of each exercise. Rest for 30 seconds; then repeat for a total of 3 to 4 rounds. Do each superset at some point throughout the day.

1 LAWNMOWER RESISTANCE BAND ROW

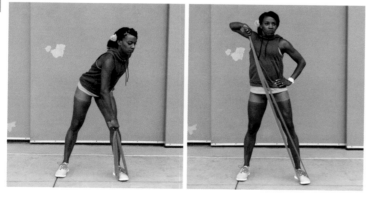

Anchor the band under one foot and hold it in the opposite hand. Pull the band up toward your shoulder, keeping your core engaged and elbow high. Return to the start position, slow and controlled. Work both sides.

CHEST PRESS

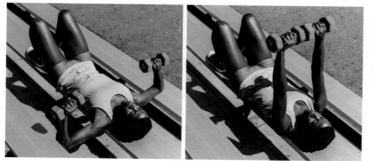

Lie on a bench, holding dumbbells straight up over your shoulders. Lower dumbbells to shoulders and press back up.

2 SINGLE-ARM DUMBBELL ROW

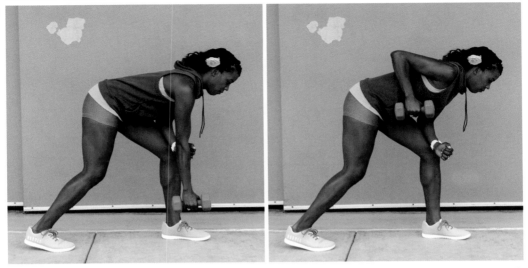

Start from a split stance, hinging forward at the hips. Hold a dumbbell in the arm opposite your forward leg and pull your elbow straight up, bringing the weight toward your torso. Keep both your back and your shoulder blades flat. Place your resting arm on the forward leg for stability. Work both sides.

 SINGLE-ARM OVERHEAD PRESS

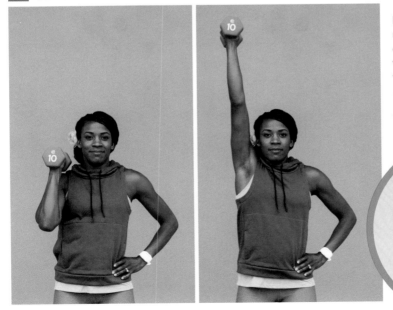

Press one weight straight up; then lower it back down to your shoulder with control. Keep your core engaged so you don't carry the load with your low back. Work both sides.

No dumbbells?

Water bottles, melons, and even filled-up canvas tote bags make great weights. Work with what you've got and remember that something is always more than nothing!

3 BAND PULL-APART

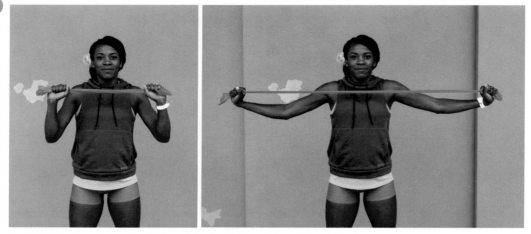

Hold the band palms out, with hands just outside of shoulder-width. Engage your core, squeeze your scapulas, and pull until your arms (and the band) are fully extended.

OVERHEAD TRICEPS EXTENSION

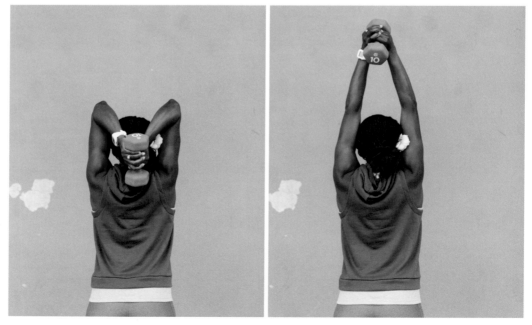

Hold the weight overhead, arms extended, and lower it with control. Keep your elbows tucked and your core strong to avoid loading your low back.

MOBILITY CIRCUIT

Here, every exercise will feel like a cross between a strength workout and a stretch, and that's what mobility is all about. Learn to move and control your body in new ways through dedicated hip, core, and shoulder drills.

▶ **Perform 8 to 12 reps of exercises 1–7 back-to-back. Rest for 30 seconds; then repeat the circuit for a total of 4 to 5 rounds. Knock out all of the rounds throughout the day.**

1 HIP CIRCLES

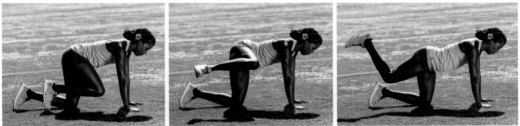

From an all-fours position, keep your core engaged as you lift your knee first out to the side, then around and behind you, and then forward to start another circle. Halfway through your reps, reverse direction. Work the other side.

≫ STRAIGHT-LEG HIP CIRCLES

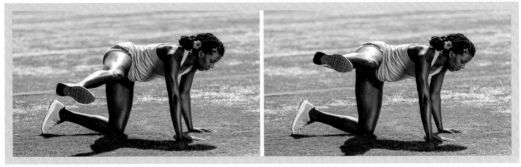

Engage your glutes to raise one leg straight out to your side. In one fluid motion, make a circle with your foot. Halfway through your reps, reverse direction. Work the other side.

2 SUPERWOMAN

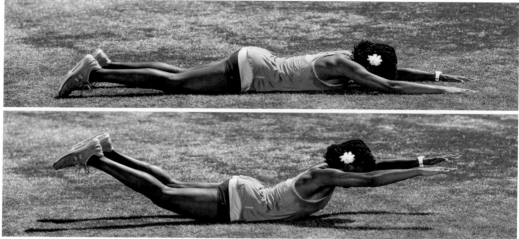

Extend your arms and engage your trunk muscles to lift your arms and legs; then lower back down with control. Back off the lift slightly if you feel the load in your low back.

3 HIP SWITCH

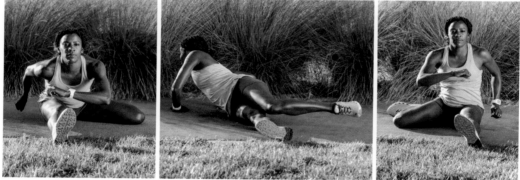

Sit with one leg extended and your other leg bent at a 90-degree angle behind you. Lean forward with the opposite arm leading the stretch. Now swing your back leg around and roll laterally into a stretch on the opposite side. Find your rhythm, moving dynamically from side to side.

4 SIDE PLANK, THREAD THE NEEDLE

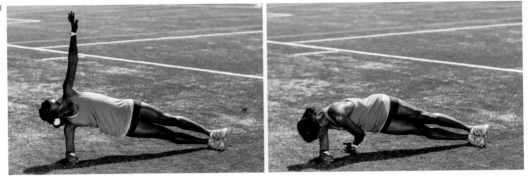

Hold a side plank. Reach your opposite arm up high, then under your torso. Track your hand with your eyes as you continue the movement. Work both sides.

5 SPLIT-LEG CROSS-TOE TOUCH

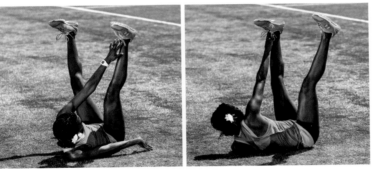

Engage your abs to raise your shoulders and reach your hand to the opposite foot; then come back down with control. Alternate sides, keeping your back flat and legs still.

» LYING CROSS-TOE TOUCH

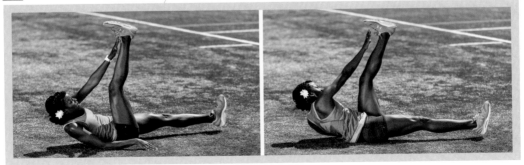

Lie down and engage your abs as you lift your heels off the ground. Reach one hand for the opposite foot as you lift your leg. Alternate sides, keeping your lower back flat and arms and legs straight.

6 WALL SLIDE

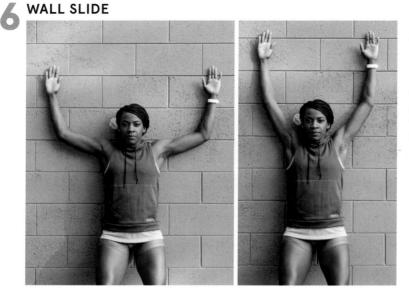

Stand with your butt, shoulders, elbows, and hands against the wall. Extend your arms up the wall, trying to limit the arch in your low back; then lower your body back down the wall.

7 LATERAL BAND WALK

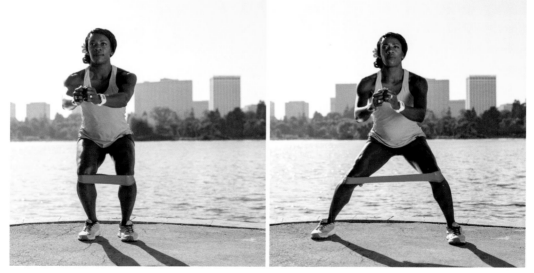

Place the band just below your knees. From a half-squat stance, step one foot out to the side and follow with the opposite foot, keeping the band taut at all times. Return in the opposite direction to work the other side.

TOTAL-BODY SUPERSETS

Each exercise in this workout will train your body from head to toe. That said, each also has its own little specialty. For example, the second exercise in each superset mimics running patterns to keep you on your running toes even when you're short on space.

▶ **Perform 8 to 12 reps of each exercise in the superset. Rest for 30 seconds; then repeat the superset for a total of 3 to 4 rounds. Make it through all of the supersets by the end of the day.**

 SUMO SQUAT WITH PRESS

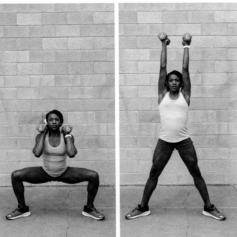

Get into a wide sumo stance, toes pointed outward and weights in front of your shoulders. Squat down and drive through your heels, pressing the weights overhead. Keep your core engaged—you shouldn't feel the load in your low back.

≫ SQUAT TO PRESS

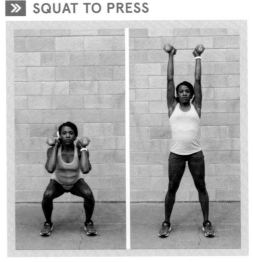

Move your feet to be shoulder-width apart, weights in front of your shoulders. Squat down and drive through your heels, pressing the weights overhead.

RUNNING JACK

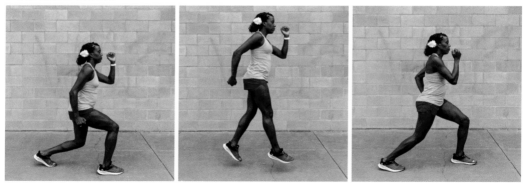

For this jack, jump with one foot forward and one back, arms moving opposite your legs.

2 DEADLIFT TO BENT-OVER ROW

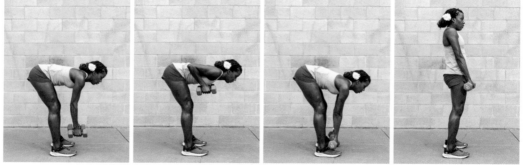

Hinge at the hips and lower the weights close to your body, until your back is parallel with the ground. Turn your palms inward. Pinch your shoulder blades together as you "row," pulling the weights up to your torso (with elbows tucked); then lower back down. Now push your ribs forward to return to standing.

JACK SQUAT

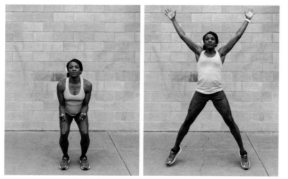

Start from a squat, arms tucked; then pop up and out into the jack position, legs and arms out. Spring from squat to jack and back without pausing.

3 PUSH-UP SIDE KNEE HIKES

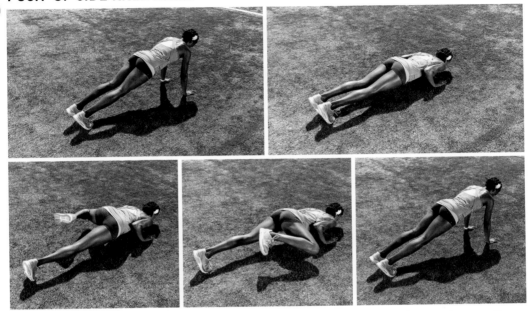

Get into a high-plank position and lower your body into a push-up. Pump your knee up to your elbow, then switch knees before pushing back up to a high plank. Keep the sequence going.

HIGH KNEES

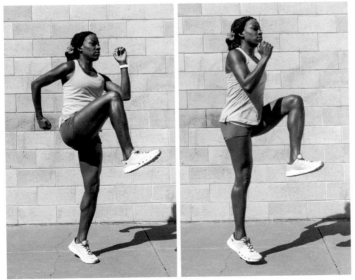

Drive one knee up, and feel the lift as you hop-skip up to the ball of your foot; alternate sides. Drive your arms in a tight stride, opposite your legs.

AGILITY DRILLS

Put everything together—strength, coordination, and mobility—with this run-centric agility workout! Remember, agility is as much mental as it is physical. Stay focused, cut your reaction time, and explode!

▶ **Do 8 to 12 reps of each exercise in the superset. Rest for 30 seconds; then repeat the superset for a total of 3 to 4 rounds. Complete them all throughout the day.**

1 A-SKIP

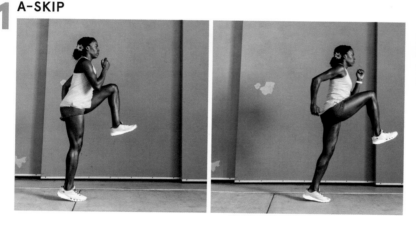

Hop-skip with high knees, swinging your arms to keep momentum.

B-SKIP

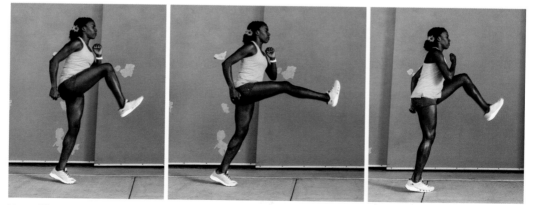

Hop-skip, engaging your glute to pull your knee up (like the A-Skip), then swing your leg forward to extension. Move your arms for momentum.

2 SIDE-TO-SIDE HOP-OVER

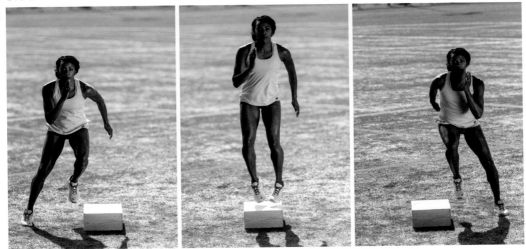

Move from side to side over the top of a step or stationary object, with a quick stutter-step at the top or midpoint. Get your arms pumping opposite your legs for added momentum.

SINGLE-LEG POWER-UP

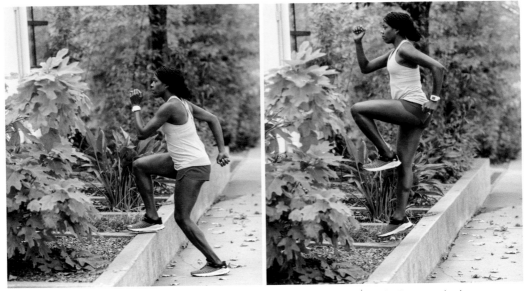

Start with one foot up on a bench or step. Drive through that leg as you explode up and raise your opposite knee toward your chest; then land soft and step back down. Keep a steady rhythm, moving your arms opposite your legs to create momentum. Work both sides.

3 X JUMP

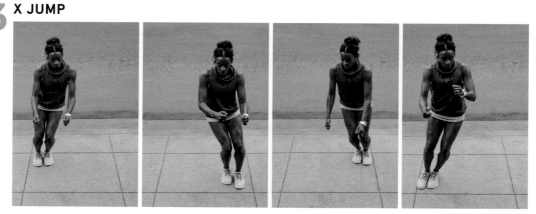

Keep your feet together as you jump from corner to corner, hitting all four corners of a square—diagonally forward, back, diagonally forward, then back to the first corner. Switch directions halfway through the rep count.

SPLIT SQUAT JUMP

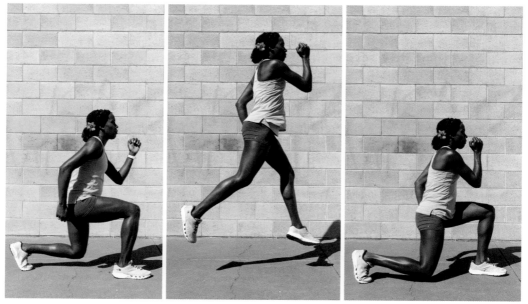

Start in a split stance and pop up. Switch your stance as you hit the height of your jump and land soft. Get your arms moving opposite your legs so you can tap that momentum.

Challenge 4

SUPPORT YOUR
RUNNING HABIT

Congrats! By now, you're in the habit of movement, and ready to add to the foundation you've built over the last three challenges. Time to run a 5K!

This month, you'll develop the ability to stick with almost-daily 30- to 45-minute workouts, get familiar with new training techniques, such as plyometrics and repeats, and use some potentially new-to-you equipment. Sweaty high fives all around!

If you feel a bit of anxiety heading into this challenge, that's okay and totally normal. Listen to your body. If the workouts in this challenge feel too long or hard, or you opened the book straight to Challenge 4, you could benefit from giving yourself an extra go-around with the first three challenges—especially Challenge 1.

So take a deep breath, trust your training, and, most importantly, get excited!

FLOWER POWER

Confidence

You are the owner of you. You 100 percent to deserve to walk with your head held high and say "Yeah, I'm the mother effin' shiiiii'" . . . because guess what? You are!

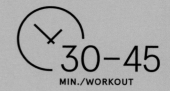

30–45
MIN./WORKOUT

5–6 days per week for *4 weeks*

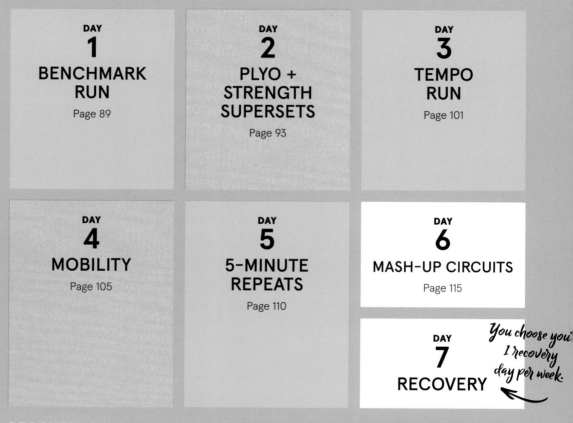

DAY
1
BENCHMARK
RUN
Page 89

DAY
2
PLYO +
STRENGTH
SUPERSETS
Page 93

DAY
3
TEMPO
RUN
Page 101

DAY
4
MOBILITY
Page 105

DAY
5
5-MINUTE
REPEATS
Page 110

DAY
6
MASH-UP CIRCUITS
Page 115

DAY
7
RECOVERY

You choose your 1 recovery day per week.

RECOVERY DAYS   If you do want to get a little recovery work in, check out the **Foam Rolling** and **Mobility** routines in the Appendix (p. 270).

EQUIPMENT   Running shoes ▪ dumbbells ▪ kettlebell ▪ 2 resistance bands (1 short, 1 long) ▪ medicine ball ▪ foam roller

For the final week
Drop the repeats on Day 5 and swap out the Mash-up Circuits for Mobility work or a day off prior to your 5K.

BENCHMARK RUN

Just like we did in Challenge 1, you will start each week of this next-level challenge by checking in with yourself! This workout will take you through a gentle warm-up, activation drills, and a 1-mile time trial. Track your results from week to week to celebrate your progress. On the last day of this challenge we'll step things up with a 5K time trial!

▶ Complete an easy 10-minute jog to get your heart rate up and muscles ready to go. Aim for an RPE of 3 to 4. Spend 1 minute with each foam rolling movement.

GLUTE ROLL

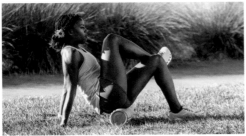

Cross one leg into a figure-4 position and roll out the glute of the stationary leg. Switch sides.

CALF ROLL

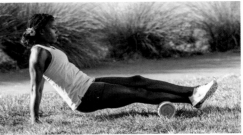

Roll out your calf muscle, using your opposite leg to go a little deeper. Roll out both sides.

UPPER-BACK ROLL

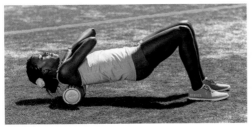

Position a foam roller under your shoulders and lift your hips. Move your feet to shift the roller up and down your back.

HIP FLEXOR ROLL

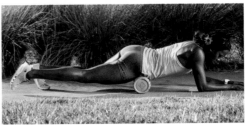

Stabilize yourself with one foot and gently roll out your hip flexor on the opposite leg. Switch sides.

▶ Do 5 to 8 reps of exercises 1–3, rest 20–30 seconds, and then repeat for a total of 2 rounds.

1 SPLIT-LEG CRUNCH

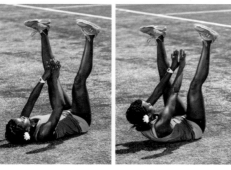

With legs extended, engage your abs to raise your shoulders and reach; then come back down with control. Keep your back flat and legs still.

⟫ SPLIT-LEG CROSS-TOE TOUCH

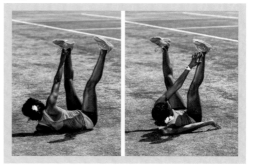

Raise your shoulders and reach your hand to the opposite foot; then come back down with control. Alternate sides, keeping your back flat and legs still.

2 ALTERNATING SUPERWOMAN

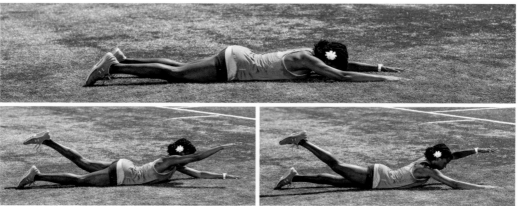

Engage your trunk muscles to lift and lower the opposing arm and leg with control; alternate sides. Back off the lift slightly if you feel the load in your low back.

3 B-SKIP

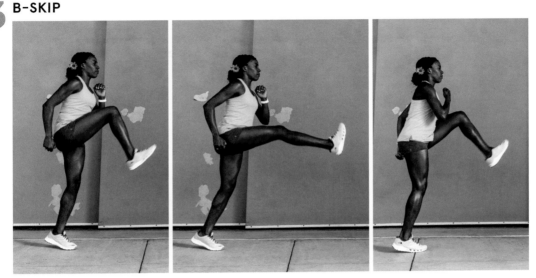

Hop-skip, engaging your glute to pull your knee up, then swing your leg forward to extension. Move your arms for momentum.

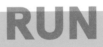

TIME TRIAL Give it all you've got! Using a running watch or following a set course, time how fast you can run 1 mile (RPE 7). Here's a tip: Track your time for the first 200m, and do your best to hold that pace. Check in every 200m if you can mentally handle it, or just check your pace on every full lap (0.25 mile).

WEEKLY PROGRESSIONS

Weeks 2–4: Try to increase your mile pace from week to week! Every second is a win!

Day 31: Today's the day for your 5K time trial! You've got this!

▶ Hold each stretch
for 5 seconds, take a
breath, and see if you
can stretch a little farther.
Do this 5–6 times, then
repeat on the other side.

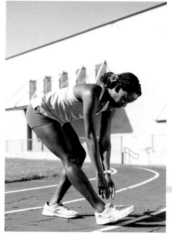

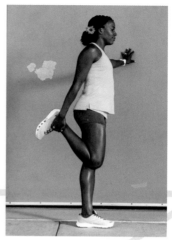

STANDING HAMSTRING STRETCH

Extend one leg just out in
front of you and let the knee
of the opposite leg bend
as you reach forward.
Try to keep your back flat.

STANDING QUAD STRETCH

Using a wall for support,
stand on one leg and pull the
opposite heel to your glute.
Press forward through your
stretched side to keep
your hips and knees square.

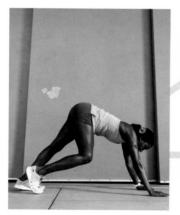

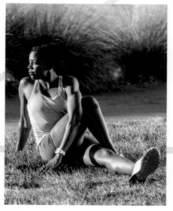

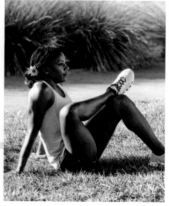

DOWNWARD DOG CALF STRETCH

Push your palms and heels
into the ground, bending one
knee at a time as you push
the opposite heel to the
ground to stretch that calf.

SEATED SPINAL ROTATION

With legs extended, cross one
leg over the other and twist
in the opposite direction,
using your arm to push your
knee in toward your chest.

SEATED GLUTE STRETCH

With knees bent, cross one
leg over the other to get into
a figure-4 position. Gently
move closer to your stationary
foot to intensify the stretch.

PLYO + STRENGTH SUPERSETS

This total-body workout starts off with explosive plyometric moves, then alternates between lower- and upper-body moves. You'll keep your heart rate elevated and build stamina right along with muscle!

WARM-UP

▶ **Spend 1 minute with each foam rolling movement.**

GLUTE ROLL

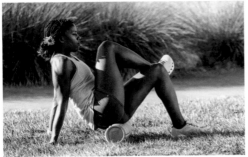

Cross one leg into a figure-4 position and roll out the glute of the stationary leg. Switch sides.

CALF ROLL

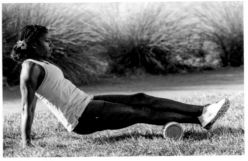

Roll out your calf muscle, using your opposite leg to go a little deeper. Roll out both sides.

UPPER-BACK ROLL

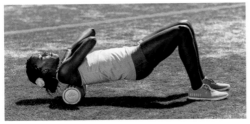

Position a foam roller under your shoulders and lift your hips. Move your feet to shift the roller up and down your back.

HIP FLEXOR ROLL

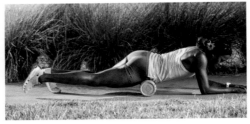

Stabilize yourself with one foot and gently roll out your hip flexor on the opposite leg. Switch sides.

▶ Do 5 to 8 reps of exercises 1–5, rest 15 seconds, and then repeat for a total of 2 rounds.

1 DONKEY KICK

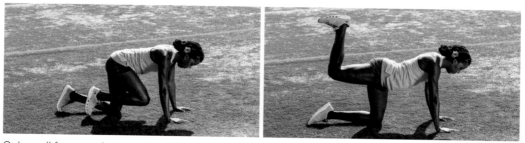

Get on all fours, and engage your glutes to raise your foot up behind you and lower it back down with control. Use your core to keep your back flat and feel the glutes burn, even on the stationary leg. Work both sides.

2 FIRE HYDRANT

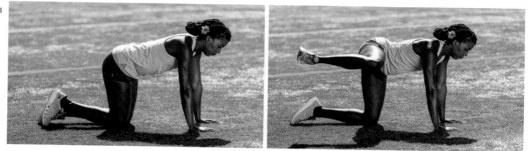

From an all-fours position lift one leg out laterally and lower it with control. Work both sides.

3 HIP CIRCLES

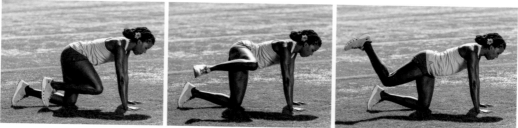

From an all-fours position, keep your core engaged as you lift your knee first out to the side, then around and behind you, and then forward to start another circle. Halfway through your reps, reverse direction. Work the other side.

4 WALK THE PLANK

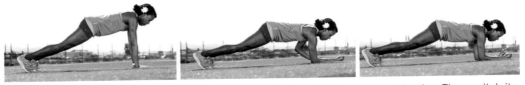

Move from a high plank to a low plank and back up again, keeping the movement going. Then switch it up to lead the up-down movement with the opposite arm. ◀ To make this easier, drop to your knees.

5 COBRA SUPERWOMAN TO LOW SUPERWOMAN

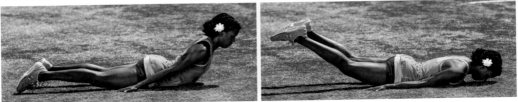

Start with your arms at your sides, palms down, and engage your trunk muscles to lift and lower your torso with control. Use your glutes to lift and lower your legs with control. Back off the lift slightly if you feel the load in your low back.

≫ SUPERWOMAN

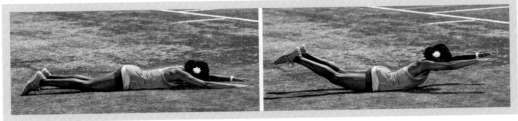

Extend your arms and engage your trunk muscles to lift your arms and legs; then lower back down with control.

WEEKLY PROGRESSIONS

Week 2: Use a 4:2:1 tempo.

Week 3: Use a 4:2:1 tempo. Reduce rest between rounds to 30 seconds.

Week 4: Use a 4:2:1 tempo. Maintain rest between rounds at 30 seconds. Increase weights (or if no others available, rep count) to reach fatigue, when you feel like you can't perform 1 more rep with proper form.

See p. 14 Count Your Tempo

▶ Complete the supersets by performing 8 to 12 reps of each exercise. Rest for 1 minute; then repeat the superset for a total of 3 rounds.

Plyos

Plyometric exercises call out your fast-twitch muscles to improve agility and quickness. Stay light on your feet when you are jumping. Don't worry if you feel slow or uncoordinated at first. Keep after it and you will get faster.

1 SPLIT SQUAT JUMP

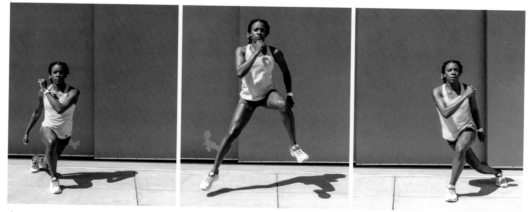

Start in a split stance and pop up. Switch your stance as you hit the height of your jump and land soft. Get your arms moving opposite your legs so you can tap that momentum.

SKATER JUMP

Jump from side to side. As you land, swing the inside leg behind you and touch down lightly before bounding back to the other side.

2 ROMANIAN DEADLIFT

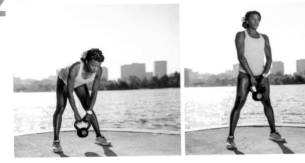

Keep your back flat and a slight bend in your knees as you hinge at the hips and lower the weight. Return to standing position in a slow, controlled movement. ▶▶ Using weight with this exercise will help build stability.

CHEST PRESS

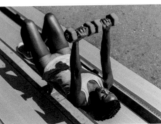

Lie on a bench, holding dumbbells straight up over your shoulders. Lower dumbbells to shoulders and press back up.

3 GOBLET SQUAT

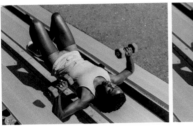

Stand with your feet just outside shoulder-width. Hold the weight at chest-height and squat down until your elbows lightly tap your thighs. Feel the weight in your heels as you come back up. Keep your core engaged and back flat.

SINGLE-ARM DUMBBELL ROW

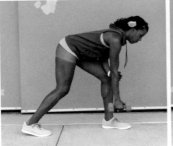
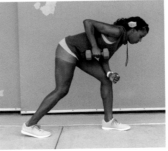

Start from a split stance, hinging forward at the hips. Hold a dumbbell in the arm opposite your forward leg and pull your elbow straight up, bringing the weight toward your torso. Keep both your back and your shoulder blades flat. Place your resting arm on the forward leg for stability. Work both sides.

4 WEIGHTED REVERSE LUNGE TO KNEE DRIVE

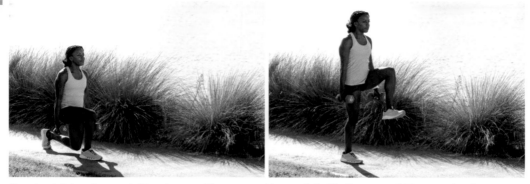

Step back into a lunge, sinking down until your quad is parallel with the ground. Then push off your back foot and bring your knee high before stepping back into a lunge again. Do all of the reps on one side, then switch. Let your legs do the work.

SINGLE-ARM OVERHEAD PRESS

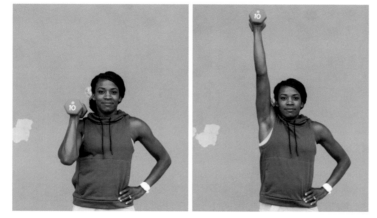

Press one weight straight up; then lower it back down to your shoulder with control. Keep your core engaged so you don't carry the load with your low back. Work both sides.

5 HAMSTRING CURL

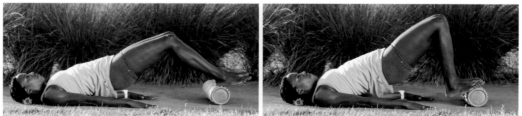

Lie on your back with the foam roller under your heels. Lift your hips up and pull your heels in until the roller reaches your toes. Continue rolling out and in.

LAWNMOWER RESISTANCE BAND ROW

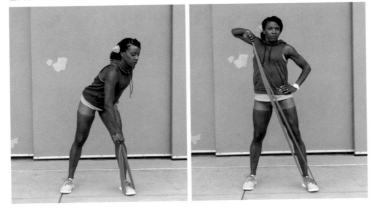

Anchor the band under one foot and hold it in the opposite hand. Pull the band up toward your shoulder, keeping your core engaged and elbow high. Return to the start position, slow and controlled. Work both sides.

6 STANDING CALF RAISE

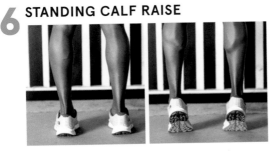

Push through the balls of your feet to raise your heels as high as possible; then lower back down with control. Hold on to a stationary object for balance if needed.

≫ SINGLE-LEG CALF RAISE

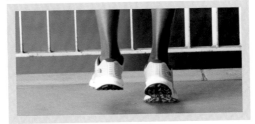

Stand on one foot and come up on your toes, then back down.

REAR DELT FLY

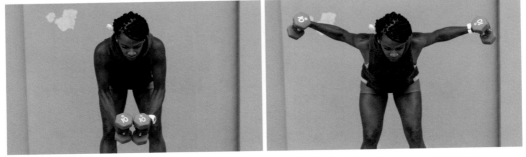

Hinge at the hips with a flat back. Squeeze your shoulder blades together to raise your arms up to shoulder height. Lower back down with control. Keep a slight bend in your elbows as you continue the movement.

▶ Hold each stretch for 5 seconds, take a breath, and see if you can stretch a little farther. Do this 5–6 times, then repeat on the other side.

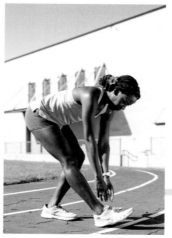

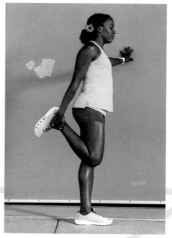

STANDING HAMSTRING STRETCH

Extend one leg just out in front of you and let the knee of the opposite leg bend as you reach forward. Try to keep your back flat.

STANDING QUAD STRETCH

Using a wall for support, stand on one leg and pull the opposite heel to your glute. Press forward through your stretched side to keep your hips and knees square.

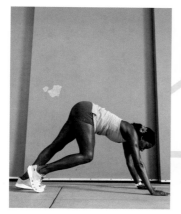

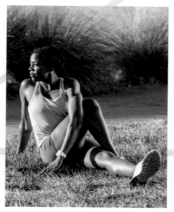

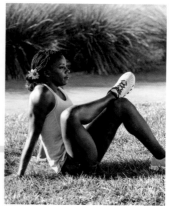

DOWNWARD DOG CALF STRETCH

Push your palms and heels into the ground, bending one knee at a time as you push the opposite heel to the ground to stretch that calf.

SEATED SPINAL ROTATION

With legs extended, cross one leg over the other and twist in the opposite direction, using your arm to push your knee in toward your chest.

SEATED GLUTE STRETCH

With knees bent, cross one leg over the other to get into a figure-4 position. Gently move closer to your stationary foot to intensify the stretch.

TEMPO RUN

Great for increasing your anaerobic threshold, tempo runs will help you run harder and faster, without hitting the infamous wall.

WARM-UP

▶ Get the blood pumping with an easy 10-minute jog. Aim for an average RPE of 3 to 4. Then spend 1 minute with each foam rolling movement.

GLUTE ROLL

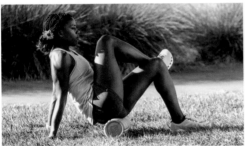

Cross one leg into a figure-4 position and roll out the glute of the stationary leg. Switch sides.

CALF ROLL

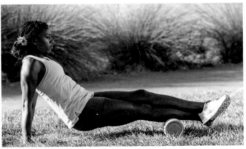

Roll out your calf muscle, using your opposite leg to go a little deeper. Roll out both sides.

UPPER-BACK ROLL

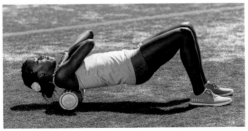

Position a foam roller under your shoulders and lift your hips. Move your feet to shift the roller up and down your back.

HIP FLEXOR ROLL

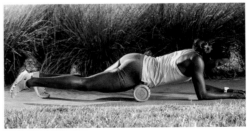

Stabilize yourself with one foot and gently roll out your hip flexor on the opposite leg. Switch sides.

▶ Do 5 to 8 reps of exercises 1–4, rest 15 seconds, and then repeat for a total of 2 rounds.

1 I, Y, AND T RAISES

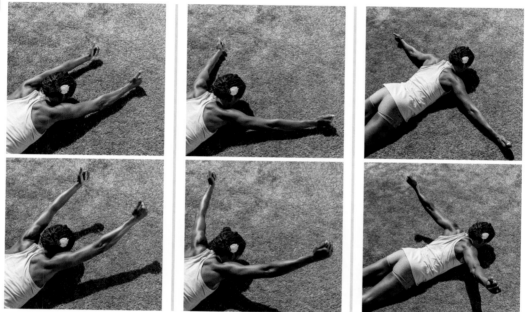

Lie down and squeeze your shoulder blades together to raise and lower your arms overhead in an "I" position, slow and controlled. Move from your shoulders, with your thumbs leading the way. Repeat to get in your Y and T raises, 5 to 8 reps of each.

2 DOUBLE HEEL SLIDE

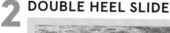
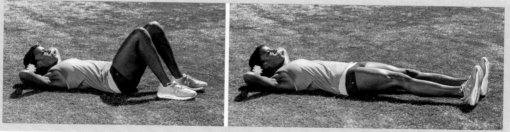

Slide both heels out and back in, keeping your core engaged and your low back flat.

3 SIDE LUNGE

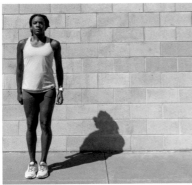
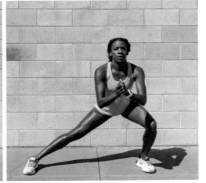

Step out to one side into a squat; then push off back to start. Work both sides.

4 SPLIT SQUAT JUMP

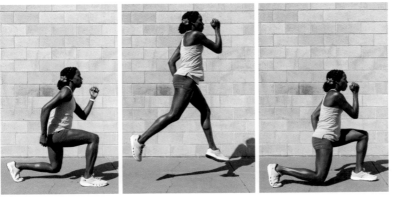

Start in a split stance and pop up. Switch your stance as you hit the height of your jump and land soft. Get your arms moving opposite your legs so you can tap that momentum.

RUN

TEMPO Run or jog for 30 minutes at a pace that would allow you to keep going for 10 more minutes . . . if you had to (RPE 5 to 6). The goal isn't to completely wipe yourself out here, but to improve your ability to listen to your body, set a pace, and stick to it!

WEEKLY PROGRESSIONS

Sure, you want to get a little faster from week to week, but since our focus is on pacing, each week, try to make your splits a little more steady than the week before. Aim to run each mile at a consistent pace rather than pushing a little too hard and having to back off your tempo pace.

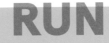

▶ Hold each stretch for 5 seconds, take a breath, and see if you can stretch a little farther. Do this 5–6 times, then repeat on the other side.

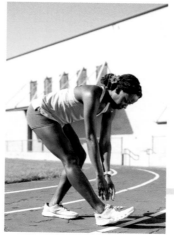

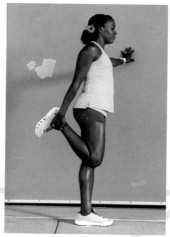

STANDING HAMSTRING STRETCH

Extend one leg just out in front of you and let the knee of the opposite leg bend as you reach forward. Try to keep your back flat.

STANDING QUAD STRETCH

Using a wall for support, stand on one leg and pull the opposite heel to your glute. Press forward through your stretched side to keep your hips and knees square.

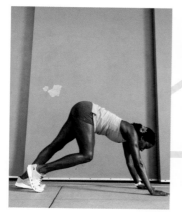

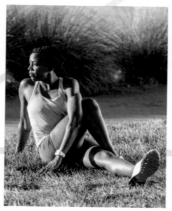

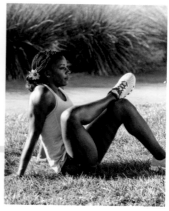

DOWNWARD DOG CALF STRETCH

Push your palms and heels into the ground, bending one knee at a time as you push the opposite heel to the ground to stretch that calf.

SEATED SPINAL ROTATION

With legs extended, cross one leg over the other and twist in the opposite direction, using your arm to push your knee in toward your chest.

SEATED GLUTE STRETCH

With knees bent, cross one leg over the other to get into a figure-4 position. Gently move closer to your stationary foot to intensify the stretch.

MOBILITY

Improve your joints' stability and range of motion for better form, performance, and injury prevention.

▶ **Spend 1 minute with each foam rolling movement.**

GLUTE ROLL

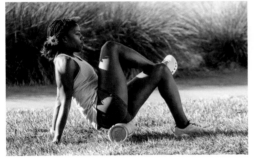

Cross one leg into a figure-4 position and roll out the glute of the stationary leg. Switch sides.

CALF ROLL

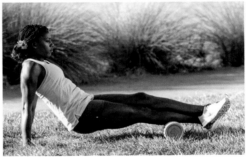

Roll out your calf muscle, using your opposite leg to go a little deeper. Roll out both sides.

UPPER-BACK ROLL

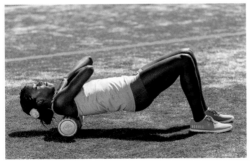

Position a foam roller under your shoulders and lift your hips. Move your feet to shift the roller up and down your back.

HIP FLEXOR ROLL

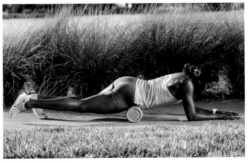

Stabilize yourself with one foot and gently roll out your hip flexor on the opposite leg. Switch sides.

▶ Do 8 to 12 reps of the exercises in each superset back-to-back. Rest for 30 seconds; then repeat for a total of 3 rounds.

1 WALL SLIDE

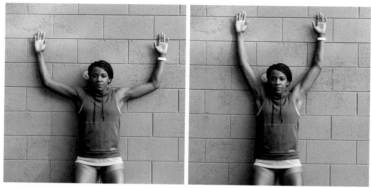

Stand with your butt, shoulders, elbows, and hands against the wall. Extend your arms up the wall, trying to limit the arch in your low back; then lower your body back down the wall.

LATERAL BAND WALK

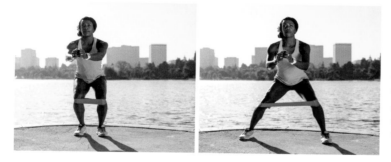

Place the band just below your knees. From a half-squat stance, step one foot out to the side and follow with the opposite foot, keeping the band taut at all times. Return in the opposite direction to work the other side.

BAND WALK

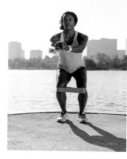
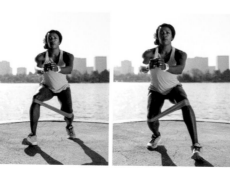

Stand with your feet shoulder-width apart and walk forward, heel-to-toe, keeping the band taut. Halfway through the reps walk backward, toe-to-heel.

2 HIP LIFT

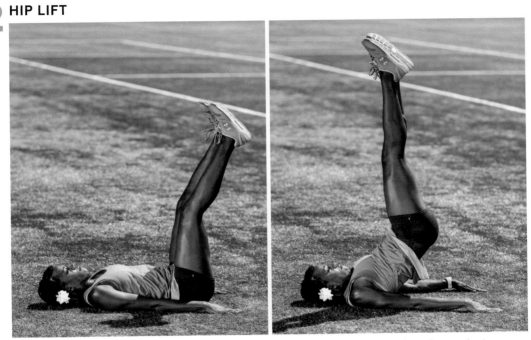

Lie on your back with your legs extended. Use your core to push your hips and reach your feet upward. Come back down with control.

» HEEL TOUCH

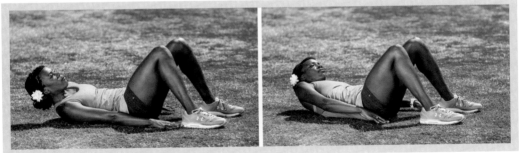

Engage your core just enough to lift your shoulders off the ground, and hold that position as you reach for your heel. Alternate side to side.

REVERSE PLANK WITH LEG LIFT

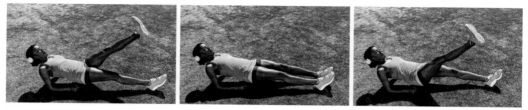

Lean back on your elbows and lift your body into plank position. Engage your core as you alternate leg lifts—only as high as you can go while holding the plank.

≫ REVERSE PLANK WITH LEG LIFT AND LATERAL EXTENSION

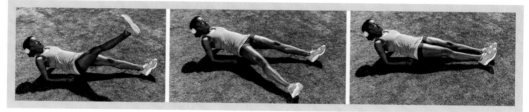

Lift one leg up, then out to the side. Continue holding the plank as you alternate sides. Engage your core as you lift one leg out and in.

3 HIP CIRCLES

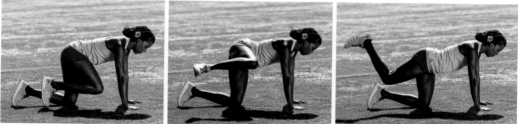

From an all-fours position, keep your core engaged as you lift your knee first out to the side, then around and behind you, and then forward to start another circle. Halfway through your reps, reverse direction. Work the other side.

I, Y, AND T RAISES

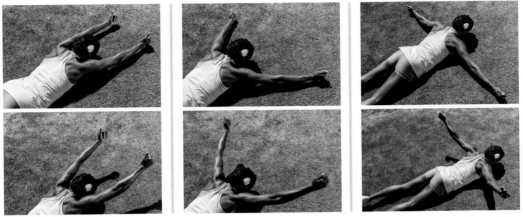

Lie down and squeeze your shoulder blades together to raise and lower your arms overhead in an "I" position, slow and controlled. Move from your shoulders, with your thumbs leading the way. Repeat to get in your Y and T raises.

 ## FORWARD LEG SWING

SIDEWAYS LEG SWING

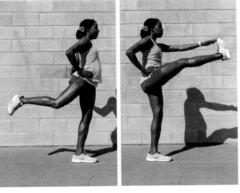

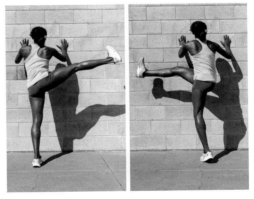

Swing one leg forward and back. Hold a wall for stability if needed. Repeat on the other side.

Face the wall and swing one leg from side to side. Work the other side.

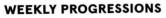

WEEKLY PROGRESSIONS

Week 2: Perform 12 to 16 reps.

Week 3: Perform 12 to 16 reps. Rest for 15 seconds.

Week 4: Perform 12 to 16 reps. Rest for 15 seconds. Perform 4 sets.

5-MINUTE REPEATS

It's time to hit it hard! Repeats are an awesome opportunity to recruit fast-twitch muscle fibers, build speed, and improve your body's ability to recover.

WARM-UP

▶ Do a 10-minute jog at RPE 3 to 4.

ACTIVATION DRILLS

▶ Do 5 to 8 reps of each exercise, resting 15 seconds between each exercise.

ROLY-POLY POWER JUMP

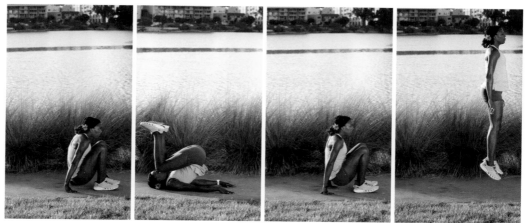

Start in a standing position, sit down, roll backward, bringing your knees to chest; then quickly roll up onto your feet and power up into a jump.

HIGH-KNEE WALL HIKES

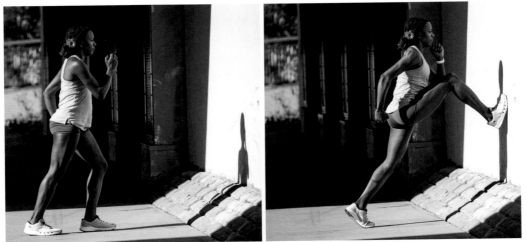

From a staggered stance swing your back leg forward to touch down on the wall as close to hip-height as possible. Swing back to reload, pumping your arms in opposition with your legs. Work both sides.

JACK SQUAT

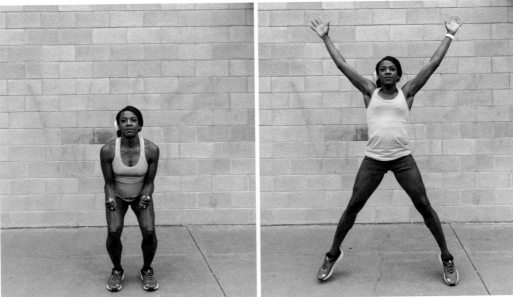

Start from a squat, arms tucked; then pop up and out into the jack position, legs and arms out. Spring from squat to jack and back without pausing.

RUN

5-MINUTE REPEATS Perform four 5-minute repeats, running at the max pace you can maintain for 5 minutes at a time (RPE 7 to 8). Between each repeat, slow to a fast walk or slow jog until your heart rate has come down; then hit that next run! Note that your rest may start at 3 minutes and progress to as little as 60–90 seconds, but keep it there so the 5-minute repeats remain a max effort.

WEEKLY PROGRESSIONS
Try to make your last repeat just as fast as your first!

CORE FINISHER

▶ Do 8 to 12 reps of exercises back-to-back. Rest for 30 seconds; then repeat for a total of 3 rounds.

LOW PLANK ▶ Hold 10–20 seconds for each set.

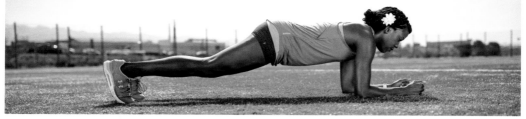

Position your elbows under your shoulders, and engage your core, holding your body in a straight line.
« To make this easier, drop to your knees.

» LOW PLANK WITH LATERAL TOE TAP

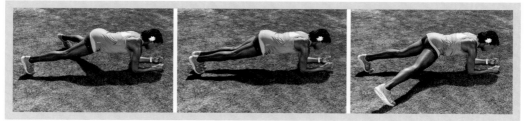

Position your elbows under your shoulders, and engage your core, holding your body in a straight line. Keep your hips steady as you alternate lateral toe taps from side to side.

SIDE PLANK ▶ Hold 10–20 seconds for each rep.

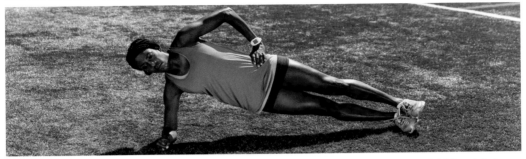

Position your elbow under your shoulder and lift your hips until your body is in a straight line. Work both sides.

 ## SIDE PLANK WITH LEG LIFT

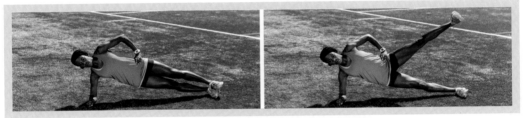

From side plank position, lift your top leg—only as high as you can go while holding the plank. Work both sides.

SUPERWOMAN

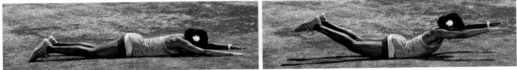

Extend your arms and engage your trunk muscles to lift your arms and legs; then lower back down with control. Back off the lift slightly if you feel the load in your low back.

⟫ TWISTING SUPERWOMAN

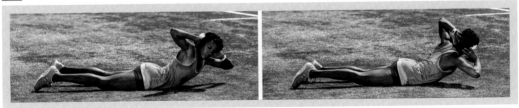

Place your hands behind your head and engage your trunk muscles to lift and twist your torso from side to side with control. Back off the lift slightly if you feel the load in your low back.

▶ Hold each stretch for 5 seconds, take a breath, and see if you can stretch a little farther. Do this 5–6 times, then repeat on the other side.

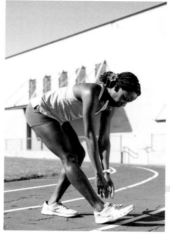

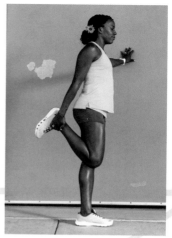

STANDING HAMSTRING STRETCH

Extend one leg just out in front of you and let the knee of the opposite leg bend as you reach forward. Try to keep your back flat.

STANDING QUAD STRETCH

Using a wall for support, stand on one leg and pull the opposite heel to your glute. Press forward through your stretched side to keep your hips and knees square.

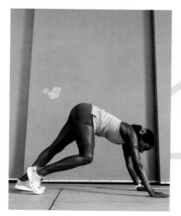

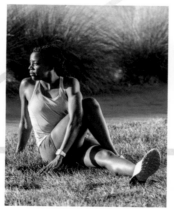

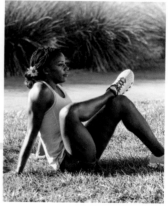

DOWNWARD DOG CALF STRETCH

Push your palms and heels into the ground, bending one knee at a time as you push the opposite heel to the ground to stretch that calf.

SEATED SPINAL ROTATION

With legs extended, cross one leg over the other and twist in the opposite direction, using your arm to push your knee in toward your chest.

SEATED GLUTE STRETCH

With knees bent, cross one leg over the other to get into a figure-4 position. Gently move closer to your stationary foot to intensify the stretch.

MASH-UP CIRCUITS

This workout puts everything together, combining some challenging running intervals with strength and agility intervals while your heart is still pumping. Hold on . . . this is the hard work that leads to big gains.

WARM-UP

▶ Get the blood pumping with an easy 10-minute jog. Aim for an average RPE of 3 to 4. Spend 1 minute with each foam rolling movement.

GLUTE ROLL

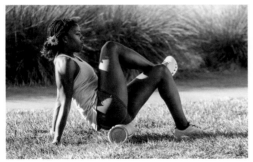

Cross one leg into a figure-4 position and roll out the glute of the stationary leg. Switch sides.

CALF ROLL

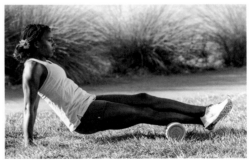

Roll out your calf muscle, using your opposite leg to go a little deeper. Roll out both sides.

UPPER-BACK ROLL

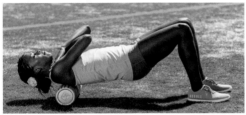

Position a foam roller under your shoulders and lift your hips. Move your feet to shift the roller up and down your back.

HIP FLEXOR ROLL

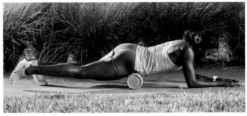

Stabilize yourself with one foot and gently roll out your hip flexor on the opposite leg. Switch sides.

RUN

MASH-UP CIRCUITS Do the following running intervals. Between each interval, do one of the circuits, performing 30 seconds of each exercise back-to-back. Rest for 2 to 3 minutes; then head into the next run interval. Repeat until you've completed all intervals and circuits. Each run interval will get shorter, giving you a chance to push the pace a little more.

1 MILE

Run 1 mile at 5K pace. If you don't know your 5K pace run at RPE 7.

SQUAT TO PRESS

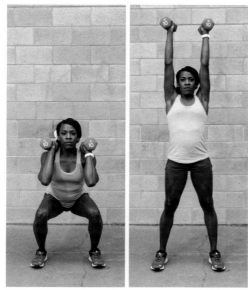

Stand with your feet shoulder-width apart, weights in front of your shoulders. Squat down and drive through your heels, pressing the weights overhead. Keep your core engaged—you shouldn't feel the load in your low back.

OVERHEAD MED BALL SLAM

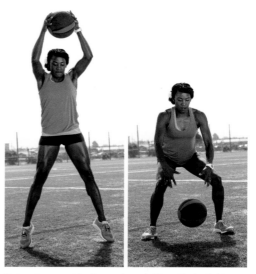

Bring the med ball overhead. Slam it straight down, catch it on the bounce, and keep on going.

INCHWORM

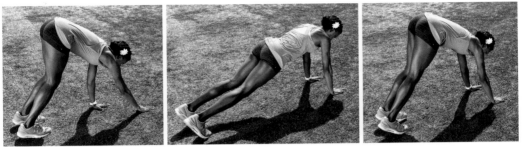

Get into a forward fold and walk your hands out into a high plank. Then walk your feet in until you are in a forward fold again. And keep on going.

>> INCHWORM WITH PUSH-UP

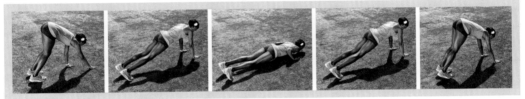

Add a push-up once you reach the high-plank position.

RUN

1,200 METERS (¾ MILE)

Pick up the pace and push effort to RPE 8.

WALKING LUNGE

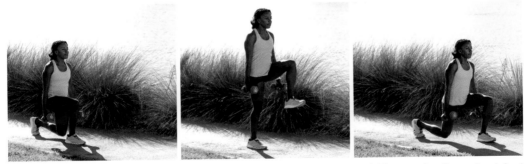

Step into a lunge, sinking down until your quad is parallel with the ground. Then push off your back foot and bring your knee high before stepping forward into a lunge on the opposite side. Let your legs do the work.

LUMBERJACK MED BALL SLAM

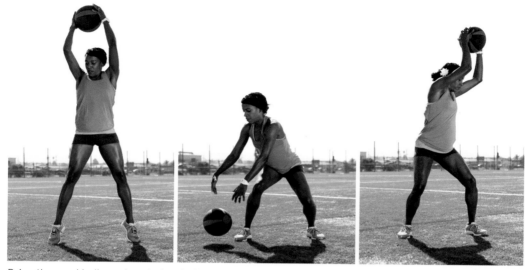

Bring the med ball overhead, slam it down to one side, catch it on the bounce, raise it overhead, and slam it down on the opposite side. Find your rhythm, moving side to side.

FORWARD LADDER SHUFFLE

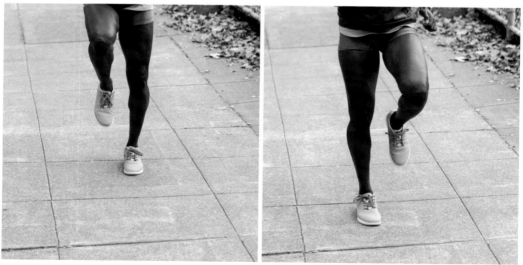

Keeping your feet under your body, spring forward onto one leg, then the other. Move forward with each step as if you're stepping between the rungs of an agility ladder. Pump your arms opposite your fast feet!

800 METERS (½ MILE)

A little faster now, RPE 8 to 9.

DEADLIFT TO BENT-OVER ROW

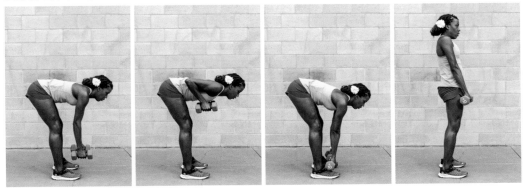

Hinge at the hips and lower the weights close to your body, until your back is parallel with the ground. Turn your palms inward. Pinch your shoulder blades together as you "row," pulling the weights up to your torso (with elbows tucked); then lower back down. Now push your ribs forward to return to standing.

OVERHEAD TRICEPS EXTENSION

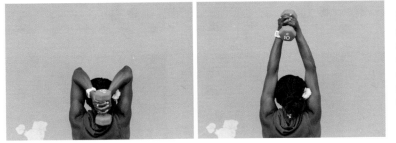

Hold the weight overhead, arms extended, and lower it with control. Keep your elbows tucked and your core strong to avoid loading your low back.

LATERAL LADDER

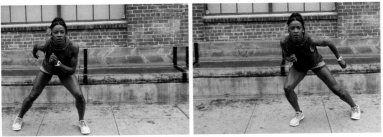

Get in a wide athletic stance and shuffle your feet from side to side, keeping your weight over the inside foot. Pump your arms for momentum and move as quickly as possible. Fast feet!

400 METERS (¼ MILE)

Give it everything you've got, RPE 9 to 10.

COOLDOWN

▶ Hold each stretch for 5 seconds, take a breath, and see if you can stretch a little farther. Do this 5–6 times, then repeat on the other side.

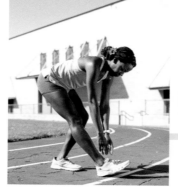

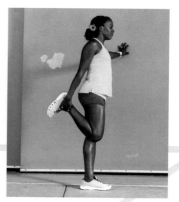

STANDING HAMSTRING STRETCH

Extend one leg just out in front of you and let the knee of the opposite leg bend as you reach forward. Try to keep your back flat.

STANDING QUAD STRETCH

Using a wall for support, stand on one leg and pull the opposite heel to your glute. Press forward through your stretched side to keep your hips and knees square.

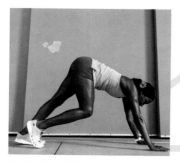

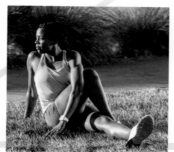

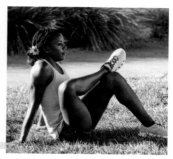

DOWNWARD DOG CALF STRETCH

Push your palms and heels into the ground, bending one knee at a time as you push the opposite heel to the ground to stretch that calf.

SEATED SPINAL ROTATION

With legs extended, cross one leg over the other and twist in the opposite direction, using your arm to push your knee in toward your chest.

SEATED GLUTE STRETCH

With knees bent, cross one leg over the other to get into a figure-4 position. Gently move closer to your stationary foot to intensify the stretch.

Challenge 5

EVERYBODY NEEDS A STRONG CORE

We tend to be pretty obsessed with our cores. Usually, our preoccupation revolves around "burning belly fat," "slimming our middles," or "toning up." I challenge you to put those goals on hold, and instead focus on making your core as strong as possible!

Nothing you do in life happens without your core muscles. Running, dancing, laughing, hugging—everything depends on a strong core. Your core supports your spine, keeps you tall and proud, and serves as the sole link between your upper and lower body. (Because what good would a set of arms and legs just flailing around be?) The core is arguably the most important part of any and every body. So, yes, you need a strong core; you deserve a strong core. And this challenge is the perfect opportunity to both celebrate and grow its strength.

Throughout the two-week challenge, you'll cycle through five different core workouts. Each will target a different function and aspect of your core, helping you learn, feel (yes, you will be sore!), and appreciate everything that your core does for you.

WEEKLY PROGRESSIONS

You'll find a lot of progressions in these workouts—so don't stop after this challenge. Make these workouts part of your regular routine.

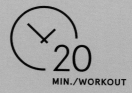

20
MIN./WORKOUT

5 days per week for *2 weeks*

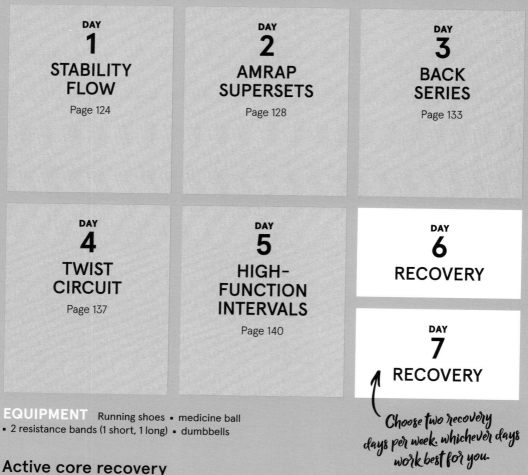

DAY 1 STABILITY FLOW Page 124	DAY 2 AMRAP SUPERSETS Page 128	DAY 3 BACK SERIES Page 133
DAY 4 TWIST CIRCUIT Page 137	DAY 5 HIGH-FUNCTION INTERVALS Page 140	DAY 6 RECOVERY
		DAY 7 RECOVERY

Choose two recovery days per week, whichever days work best for you.

EQUIPMENT Running shoes ▪ medicine ball ▪ 2 resistance bands (1 short, 1 long) ▪ dumbbells

Active core recovery

In real life, your core never gets an "off" day. So, if you want to keep it active on your recovery days (which you can and should schedule when you feel you need them!), opt for performing gentle exercises until you hit an RPE of 4 to 5. Doing so will keep your core active and blood circulating to help facilitate recovery. Rolling your upper back and the seated spinal rotation stretch feel amazing.

TAKE CARE OF YOUR CORE

Crunches have fallen out of favor in recent years. We know that crunches can cause more harm than good, mostly due to incorrect form. To support your spine and improve your core strength, you need to mix up your moves and move right. These tips apply to all of the exercises in this challenge, and any other time you are told to "engage your core."

▶ Activate your transverse abdominus by breathing out and down toward your pelvic floor.

▶ Breathe throughout the exercise: Exhale as you contract the muscles; inhale as you recover or release.

▶ Keep your movement controlled: Engage your core to move rather than pulling on your neck or otherwise trying to create momentum.

▶ Stack your spine: Don't allow your abdomen to "bulge" or "dome" to complete the movement.

Training your core with *diastasis recti*

Unfortunately, for many women, abdominal injury is a way of life. *Diastasis recti*, a separation of the rectus abdominis (six pack) muscle, commonly occurs during pregnancy as the abdomen makes room for the growing baby, and it can comprise core strength as well as increase the risk of pelvic pain and incontinence for years to come. Fortunately, returning the core to healthy function is totally possible through training.

Still, not every great core exercise (even if it's in this challenge) is great for women with DR. Trunk-flexion and elevated prone exercises are typically no-nos for anyone healing after pregnancy. Trunk-flexion exercises include the crunch, crunch twist, and anything that involves a "crunch" or "sit-up" component. Prone exercises include basically any move in which your belly hangs down, including the mountain climber, inchworm, and even exercises performed on all fours. All can put pressure on the rectus abdominis, encouraging any separation or weakness in the muscles to grow, rather than decrease.

So, if and when you run across those exercises throughout the following workouts, go ahead and either skip the move or sub it out with a DR-friendly core exercise, such as the dead bug, double or alternating heel slide, or lying scissor kick. (You'll also want to forgo the Twist Circuit on Day 4.) Also, please consider working with a physiotherapist who can prescribe the best individual rehab routine for you. Your core deserves all the care you can give it!

Every body is a beach body

Do you have a body? Are you going to the beach with it? Then you have a beach body! The saying "everybody has a beach body" inspired this challenge and inspires me to more fully appreciate my body, regardless of what I see in the mirror. It's totally okay to want to change your physical appearance, but it's important to remember that our actions are our truest reflection of self.

STABILITY FLOW

A stable, athletic core protects your spine while also enabling a more efficient connection between your upper and lower body so you can generate more total-body power.

▶ Perform 8 to 12 reps of exercises 1–6 in the circuit, rest for 1 minute, and repeat for a total of 3 rounds. Try to treat this sequence like a flow, moving seamlessly from one exercise to the next. Pretend that you're in a yoga class!

1 WALK THE PLANK

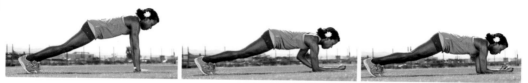

Move from a high plank to a low plank and back up again, keeping the movement going. Then switch it up to lead the up-down movement with the opposite arm. ◄ To make this easier, drop to your knees.

≫ PUSH-UP SIDE KNEE HIKES

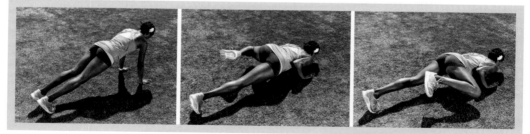

From a high-plank position, lower your body into a push-up. Pump your knee up to your elbow, then switch knees before pushing back up to a high plank. Keep the sequence going.

Mindfulness

In the everyday hustle it is easy to think that the world is conspiring against you . . . and it's personal. The weight of all of your problems, anxiety, and worry gets in the way of the bigger picture. You find yourself running on empty and focused on self-preservation, which can negatively impact your goals and also inhibit others from being able to manifest theirs. Take the opportunity to look around and notice that you are not the only one trying to succeed today. You are not alone in the struggle—it's part of being human. Reset your own intentions and thoughts against the backdrop of the bigger picture. Mindfulness is an incredibly effective way to practice self-care—it fills your tank so you can outrun whatever the day throws at you.

2 BEAR CRAWL

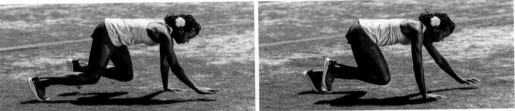

Come to your hands and the balls of your feet, and step forward with one hand and the opposite foot; then step with the opposing hand and foot. Keep your core engaged, back flat, and butt down. Halfway through the reps, move backward.

» INCHWORM

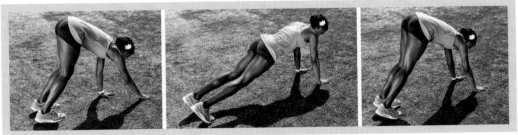

Get into a forward fold and walk your hands out into a high plank. Then walk your feet in until you are in a forward fold again. And keep on going.

3 SIDE PLANK ▶ Hold 10–20 seconds for each set.

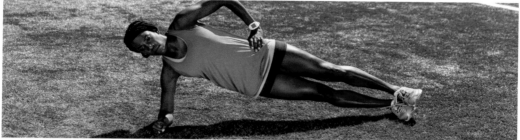

Position your elbow under your shoulder and lift your hips until your body is in a straight line. Work both sides.

≫ SIDE PLANK WITH HIP DIP

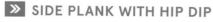

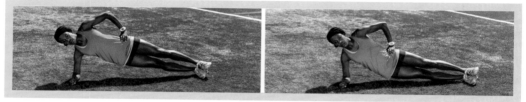

From a side plank, drop your hips down toward the ground and raise them back up into alignment. Work both sides.

4 REVERSE PLANK ▶ Hold 20–30 seconds for each set.

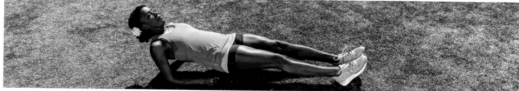

Lean back onto your elbows and engage your glutes, core, and back to hold your body in a straight line.

≫ REVERSE PLANK WITH LEG LIFT AND LATERAL EXTENSION

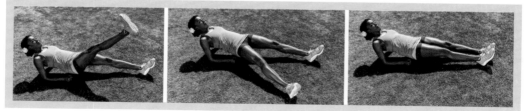

Lift one leg up, then out to the side. Continue holding the plank as you alternate sides. Engage your core as you lift one leg out and in.

5 ALTERNATING HEEL SLIDE

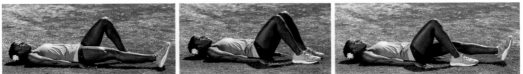

Lie down with your core engaged and your lower back flat on the ground. Slide your heel out and back in. Alternate sides.

» DOUBLE HEEL SLIDE

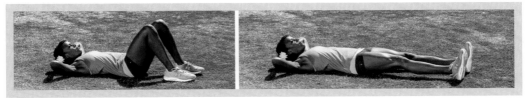

Slide both heels out and back in, keeping your core engaged and your low back flat.

6 LYING SCISSOR KICK

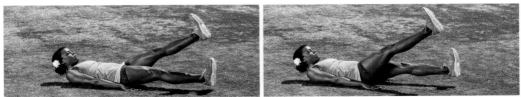

Engage your core, holding your shoulders and legs just off the ground as you "scissor" your legs up, then back down. Keep your low back flat on the ground.

» HIP LIFT

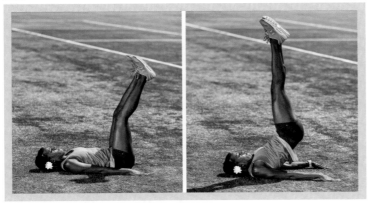

Use your core to push your hips and reach your feet upward. Come back down with control.

AMRAP SUPERSETS

Hit all 360 degrees of your core with these body-weight supersets.

▶ **Perform each exercise in the superset for as many reps as possible (AMRAP) in 30 seconds, rest for 45 to 60 seconds, and repeat for a total of 3 rounds. Complete all supersets.**

1 PUSH-UP

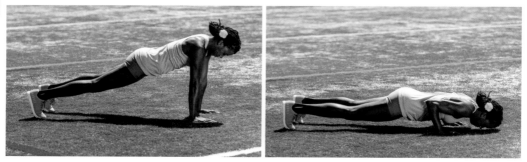

With your hands under your shoulders, squeeze your back, abs, and glutes to hold your body in a straight line. Lower your body to the ground, keeping your elbows tucked; then press back up.
« To make this easier, widen your feet.

» PUSH-UP WITH LEG LIFT

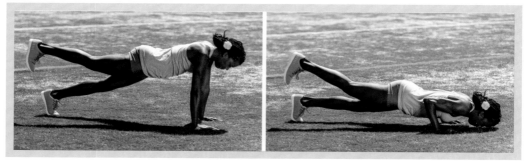

From a high-plank position, raise one leg and lower your body down, elbows tucked in, and back up. Alternate sides.

DEAD BUG

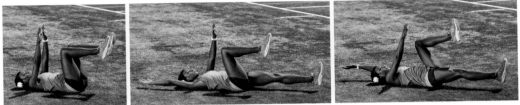

Get set with your low back flat on the ground, arms extended up, knees bent. Now move your opposing arm and leg to reach long while you move the opposite hand toward your knee. Keep alternating the movement, slow and controlled.

2 **LOW PLANK** ▷ Hold 30 seconds for each set.

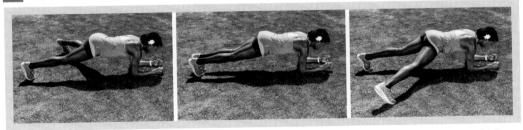

Position your elbows under your shoulders, and engage your core, holding your body in a straight line. ◀ To make this easier, drop to your knees.

≫ LOW PLANK WITH LATERAL TOE TAP

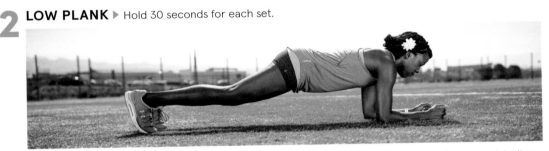

Position your elbows under your shoulders, and engage your core, holding your body in a straight line. Keep your hips steady as you alternate lateral toe taps from side to side.

SPLIT-LEG CRUNCH

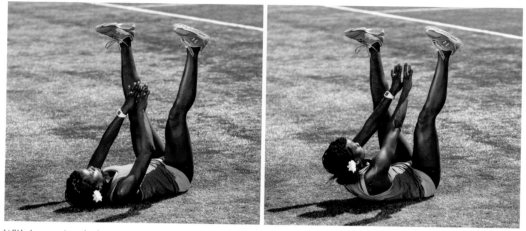

With legs extended, engage your abs to raise your shoulders and reach; then come back down with control. Keep your back flat and legs still.

» V-UP

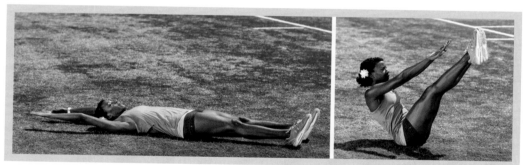

Extend your arms overhead and engage your core as you lift your legs and reach up and forward, toward your feet. Come back down with control. Keep your arms, legs, and back as straight as possible.

3 LYING CROSS-OVER SCISSOR KICK

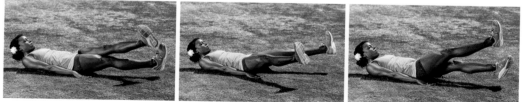

Engage your core, holding your shoulders and legs just off the ground as you "scissor" your legs over, then under. Keep your low back flat on the ground.

SIDE PLANK WITH LEG LIFT

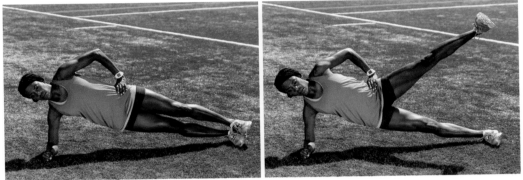

Position your elbow under your shoulder and lift your hips until your body is in a straight line. Now lift your top leg—only as high as you can go while holding the plank. Work both sides. ◀ To make this easier, do a Side Plank with Hip Dip.

 ## COBRA SUPERWOMAN

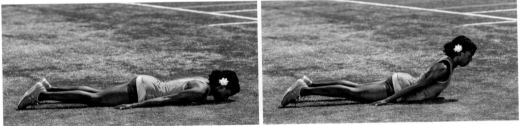

Start with your arms at your sides, palms down, and engage your trunk muscles to lift and lower your torso with control. Back off the lift slightly if you feel the load in your low back.

» SUPERWOMAN

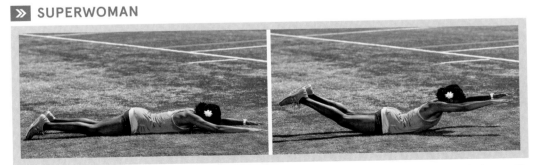

Extend your arms and engage your trunk muscles to lift your arms and legs; then lower back down with control. Back off the lift slightly if you feel the load in your low back.

I, Y, AND T RAISES

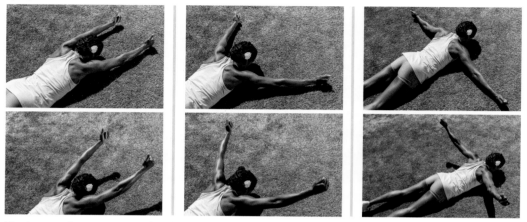

Lie down and squeeze your shoulder blades together to raise and lower your arms overhead in an "I" position, slow and controlled. Move from your shoulders, with your thumbs leading the way. Repeat to get in your Y and T raises.

5 BEAR CRAWL

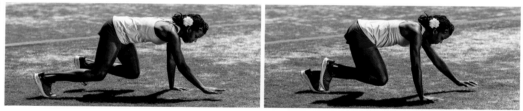

Come to your hands and the balls of your feet, and step forward with one hand and the opposite foot; then step with the opposing hand and foot. Keep your core engaged, back flat, and butt down. Halfway through the reps, move backward.

SPLIT-LEG CROSS-TOE TOUCH

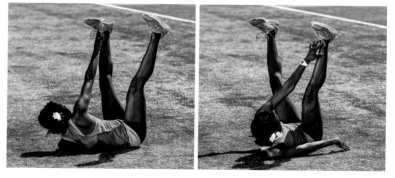

Engage your abs to raise your shoulders and reach your hand to the opposite foot; then come back down with control. Alternate sides, keeping your back flat and legs still.

BACK SERIES

The core is way more than your abs! Your posterior chain (a.k.a. backside of your body) is actually a huge portion of your core. One of the main jobs of the glutes is to stabilize your pelvis at the base of your spine. Meanwhile, muscles run along your spine like scaffolding to keep it strong, and your mid- and upper-back muscles keep you from walking around hunched over all of the time.

▶ **Perform 12 to 16 reps of each exercise in the superset, rest for 1 minute, and then perform the next superset. Complete all 4 supersets in the series.**

1 REVERSE PLANK ▶ Hold 20–30 seconds for each set.

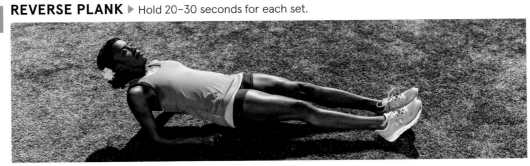

Lean back onto your elbows and engage your glutes, core, and back to hold your body in a straight line.

REVERSE PLANK WITH LEG LIFT

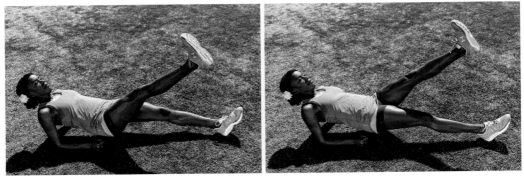

Engage your core as you alternate leg lifts—only as high as you can go while holding the plank.

REVERSE PLANK WITH LATERAL EXTENSION

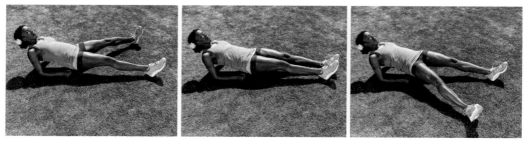

Lift one leg out and in. Alternate sides.

2 DONKEY KICK

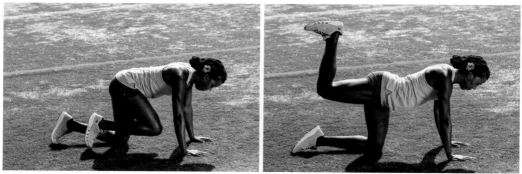

Get on all fours, and engage your glutes to raise your foot up behind you and lower it back down with control. Use your core to keep your back flat and feel the glutes burn, even on the stationary leg. Work both sides.

FIRE HYDRANT

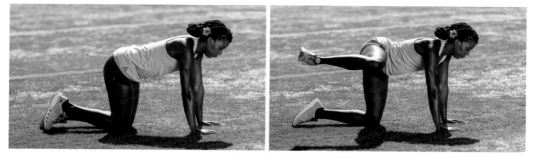

Lift one leg out laterally and lower it with control. Work both sides. ❯❯ Add a band for a bigger challenge.

HIP CIRCLES

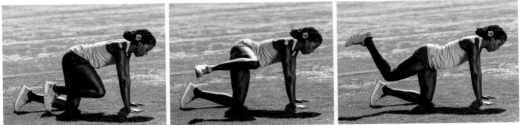

From an all-fours position, keep your core engaged as you lift your knee first out to the side, then around and behind you, and then forward to start another circle. Halfway through your reps, reverse direction. Work the other side.

3 I RAISE

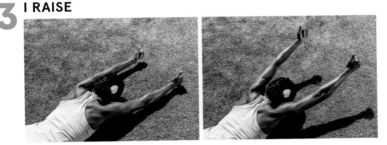

Lie down and squeeze your shoulder blades together to raise and lower your arms overhead in an "I" position, slow and controlled. Move from your shoulders, with your thumbs leading the way.

Y RAISE

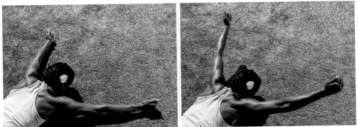

Now raise and lower your arms in a "Y" position, slow and controlled. Move from your shoulders, with your thumbs leading the way.

T RAISE

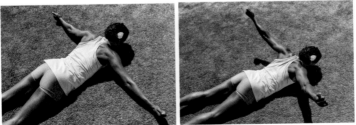

Finally, raise and lower your arms in a "T" position, slow and controlled. Move from your shoulders, with your thumbs leading the way.

>> Add light dumbbells to this superset for an added challenge.

4 COBRA SUPERWOMAN

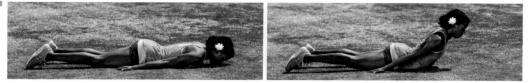

Start with your arms at your sides, palms down, and engage your trunk muscles to lift and lower your torso with control. Back off the lift slightly if you feel the load in your low back.

LOW SUPERWOMAN

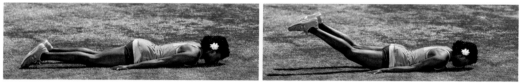

Lift and lower your legs with control.

SUPERWOMAN

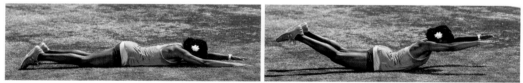

Extend your arms overhead and lift your arms and legs; then lower back down with control.

ALTERNATING SUPERWOMAN

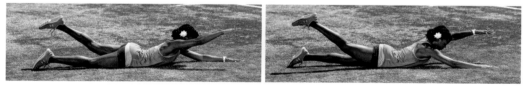

Lift and lower the opposing arm and leg with control; alternate sides.

TWISTING SUPERWOMAN

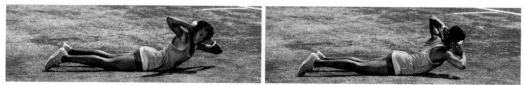

Place your hands behind your head and lift and twist your torso from side to side with control.

TWIST CIRCUIT

One awesome, often overlooked function of the core is to rotate, twist, and bend your torso from side to side. Train that ability (not to mention, your obliques) with this super-twisty workout.

▶ **Perform each exercise until you hit an RPE of 8 out of 10. Rest for 30 seconds; then repeat the circuit for a total of 3 rounds.**

1 LYING CROSS-TOE TOUCH

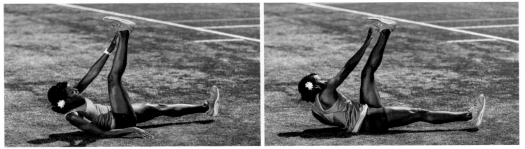

Lie down and engage your abs as you lift your heels off the ground. Reach one hand for the opposite foot as you lift your leg. Alternate sides, keeping your lower back flat and arms and legs straight.

2 SIDE PLANK, THREAD THE NEEDLE

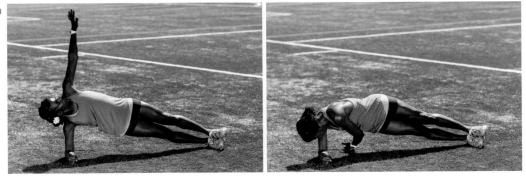

Hold a side plank. Reach your opposite arm up high, then under your torso. Track your hand with your eyes as you continue the movement. Work both sides.

3 SPLIT-LEG CROSS-TOE TOUCH

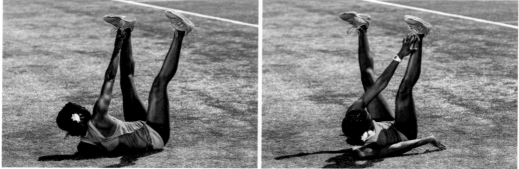

Engage your abs to raise your shoulders and reach your hand to the opposite foot; then come back down with control. Alternate sides, keeping your back flat and legs still.

4 TWISTING MOUNTAIN CLIMBER

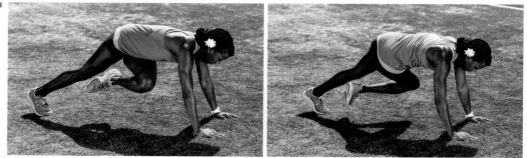

From high-plank position, bring your knee in toward the opposite elbow; alternate from side to side.

5 BICYCLE CRUNCH

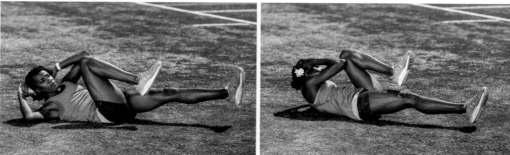

Engage your core as you pull your elbow and the opposite knee toward each other, alternating side to side.

6 HEEL TOUCH

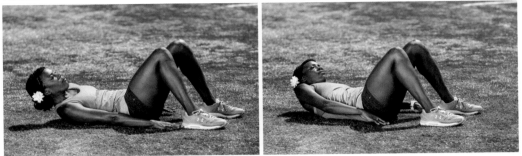

Engage your core just enough to lift your shoulders off the ground, and hold that position as you reach for your heel. Alternate side to side.

7 CRUNCH TWIST

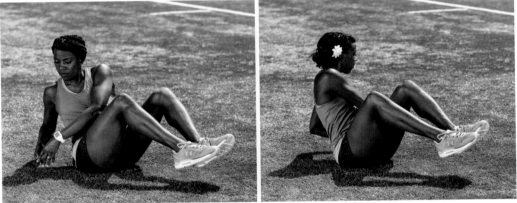

Engage your core and lift your feet off the ground, balancing on your butt. Rotate your torso as you twist from side to side, tracking your hands with your eyes.

HIGH-FUNCTION INTERVALS

Today is all about hitting the core in fun, functional ways that you may have never even thought of before. Like with single-side exercises! Yep, when loading one side of your body at a time, it's up to your core to keep you from falling over!

▶ Perform each exercise in the superset for 30 seconds, rest for 30 seconds, and then repeat the superset for a total of 4 rounds.

1 OVERHEAD MED BALL SLAM

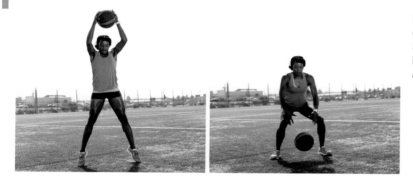

Bring the med ball overhead. Slam it straight down, catch it on the bounce, and keep on going.

LUMBERJACK MED BALL SLAM

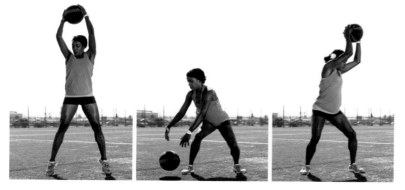

Bring the med ball overhead, slam it down to one side, catch it on the bounce, raise it overhead, and slam it down on the opposite side. Find your rhythm, moving side to side.

2 SINGLE-ARM OVERHEAD PRESS

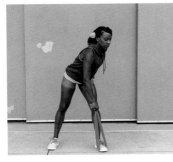
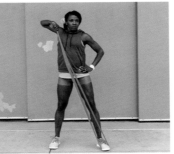

Press one weight straight up; then lower it back down to your shoulder with control. Keep your core engaged so you don't carry the load in your low back. Repeat on the other side.

LAWNMOWER RESISTANCE BAND ROW

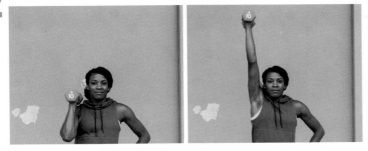

Anchor the band under one foot and hold it in the opposite hand. Pull the band up toward your shoulder, keeping your core engaged and elbow high. Return to the start position, slow and controlled. Work both sides.

3 SINGLE-ARM DUMBBELL ROW

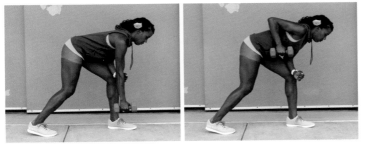

Start from a split-leg stance, hinging forward at the hips. Hold a dumbbell in the arm opposite your forward leg and pull your elbow straight up, bringing the weight toward your torso. Keep both your back and your shoulder blades flat. Work both sides.

CHEST PRESS, ALTERNATING

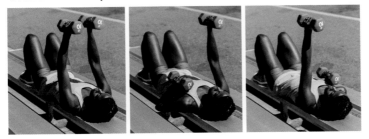

Lie on a bench, holding dumbbells straight up over your shoulders. Lower one dumbbell to your shoulder and press back up as you lower the opposite dumbbell.

Challenge 6

STIR-CRAZY CIRCUITS

We all get a little stir-crazy! Maybe you're pulling long hours in a cramped cubicle. Maybe you're stuck at home with a sick kid, spouse, or fur baby. Perhaps you spend your weeks hopping between tiny hotel rooms and even-tinier airplane seats. Or, the weather has changed your plans.

It's in times like these that our brains and bodies need movement most, but it's also exactly when we are least likely to exercise.

Trust me, I've been there. Both as the "crazed motionless" woman and the one who's like, "give me a few feet of floor space, and I can do anything!"

This workout challenge is all about enjoying movement no matter what is keeping you cooped up. It's two weeks in length, but you can expand or shrink it to fit your needs. You can even fit in a workout when you get stuck at the office!

Every workout is designed to support your running success, focusing on run-specific movements and drills, high-rep endurance exercises, and the mobility work you now know and love.

So take a deep breath and get ready to feel a whole lot less crazy!

Not there yet?

If you are doing these challenges in order, you are getting stronger, and that's why I'm throwing down some harder moves. Look for exercise modifications with this symbol ◁ to dial back the intensity.

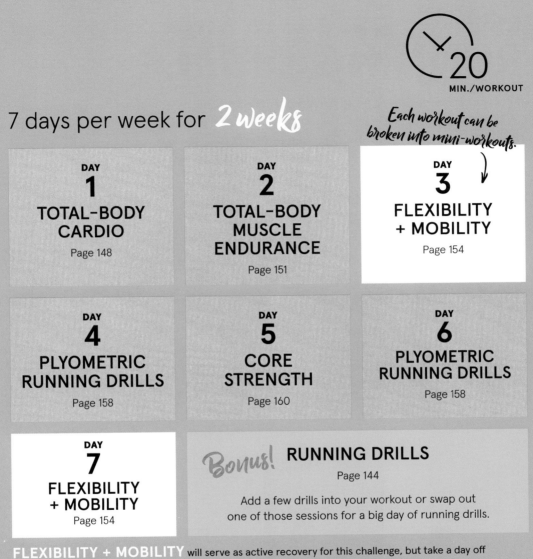

7 days per week for *2 weeks*

20
MIN./WORKOUT

Each workout can be broken into mini-workouts.

DAY
1
TOTAL-BODY CARDIO
Page 148

DAY
2
TOTAL-BODY MUSCLE ENDURANCE
Page 151

DAY
3
FLEXIBILITY + MOBILITY
Page 154

DAY
4
PLYOMETRIC RUNNING DRILLS
Page 158

DAY
5
CORE STRENGTH
Page 160

DAY
6
PLYOMETRIC RUNNING DRILLS
Page 158

DAY
7
FLEXIBILITY + MOBILITY
Page 154

Bonus! **RUNNING DRILLS**
Page 144

Add a few drills into your workout or swap out one of those sessions for a big day of running drills.

FLEXIBILITY + MOBILITY will serve as active recovery for this challenge, but take a day off if you need it.

EQUIPMENT   Running shoes • 2 resistance bands (1 short, 1 long)

Short on time?

That's totally okay! Because all the workouts in this challenge are made up of body-weight circuits, you have the option of performing all the moves one time through, going on about your day, and then repeating the circuit in batches as you have time. A few minutes here and there add up! Bonus: If you're cooped up and feeling stir-crazy, a mini-workout every few hours can help you regain your sanity!

Bonus!
RUNNING DRILLS

If you have the option to head outside or jump on the treadmill for a short run, that's great! But if you don't, having some run-specific drills in your back pocket can help you feel like the runner you are in record time. These are my favorites.

> Do 12–16 reps or 30-second intervals. Fit in sets as time allows.

HIGH KNEES

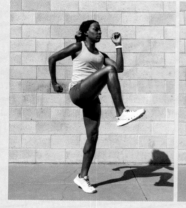 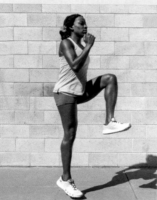

Drive one knee up, and feel the lift as you hop-skip up to the ball of your foot; alternate sides. Drive your arms in a tight stride, opposite your legs.

SPLIT SQUAT JUMP

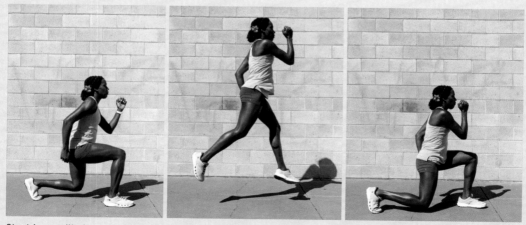

Start in a split stance and pop up. Switch your stance as you hit the height of your jump and land soft. Get your arms moving opposite your legs so you can tap that momentum.

SKATER JUMP

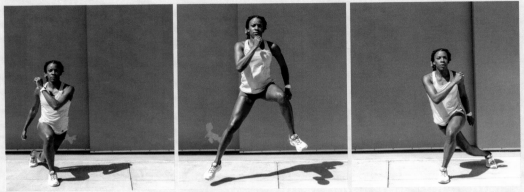

Jump from side to side. As you land, swing the inside leg behind you and touch down lightly before bounding back to the other side.

SINGLE-LEG DEADLIFT TO KNEE DRIVE

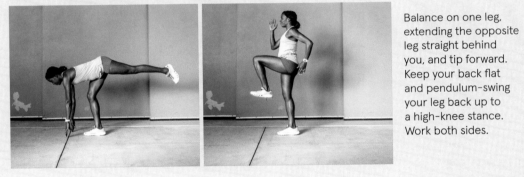

Balance on one leg, extending the opposite leg straight behind you, and tip forward. Keep your back flat and pendulum-swing your leg back up to a high-knee stance. Work both sides.

SIDE SHUFFLE

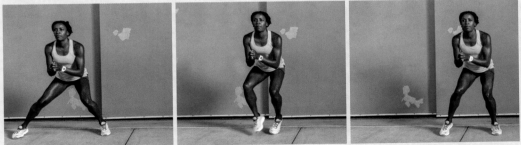

Squat slightly and shuffle with fast feet in one direction; then return the other direction. ⏩ Hold a med ball.

A-SKIP

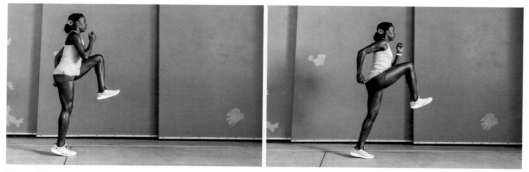

Hop-skip with high knees, swinging your arms to keep momentum.

B-SKIP

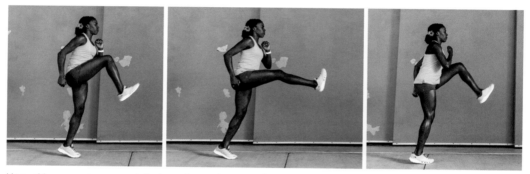

Hop-skip, engaging your glute to pull your knee up (like the A-Skip), then swing your leg forward to extension. Move your arms for momentum.

JUMP ROPE

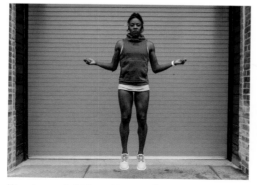

Keeping a slight bend in your knees, drive through the balls of your feet to bounce up and down as if you're jumping rope.

SINGLE-LEG JUMP ROPE

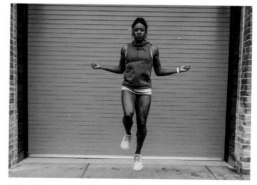

Standing on one leg and keeping a slight bend in your knee, drive through the ball of your foot to bounce up and down. Switch legs.

X JUMP

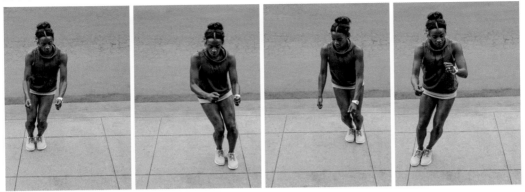

Keep your feet together as you jump from corner to corner, hitting all four corners of a square—diagonally forward, back, diagonally forward, then back to the first corner. Switch directions halfway through the rep count.

LATERAL LADDER

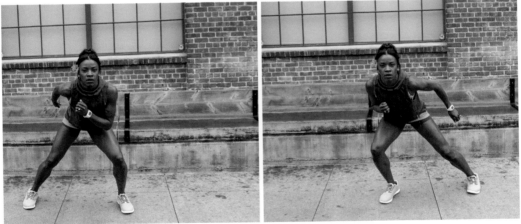

Get in a wide athletic stance and shuffle your feet from side to side, keeping your weight over the inside foot. Pump your arms for momentum and move as quickly as possible. Fast feet!

TOTAL-BODY CARDIO

This fast-moving circuit will stoke your heart rate and build aerobic capacity, translating to faster, more efficient runs, improved cardiovascular health, and easier climbs up subway stairs.

▶ Do each exercise for 30 seconds with as little rest as possible between moves. Rest for 1 minute between rounds if performing them back-to-back. Crush a total of 3 to 4 rounds throughout the day.

1 PUSH-UP SIDE KNEE HIKES

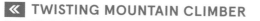

Get into a high-plank position and lower your body into a push-up. Pump your knee up to your elbow, then switch knees before pushing back up to a high plank. Keep the sequence going.

« TWISTING MOUNTAIN CLIMBER

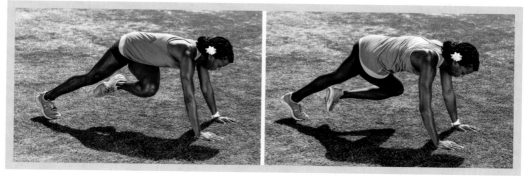

From high-plank position, bring your knee in toward the opposite elbow; alternate from side to side.

2 SINGLE-LEG JUMP ROPE

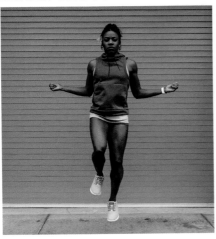

Standing on one leg and keeping a slight bend in your knee, drive through the ball of your foot to bounce up and down as if you're jumping rope. Switch legs.

3 SIDE LUNGE TO KNEE DRIVE

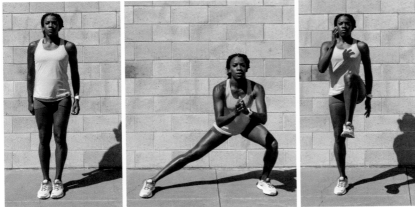

Step out to one side into a squat; then push up into a sprinter position, knee high. Work both sides.

FLOWER POWER

Visualization

Seeing isn't believing. Maybe this is reassuring because your goals are still a glimmer off in the distance. Believing starts with allowing yourself to visualize victory and success—what it looks like and feels like. This sets up your psyche to better accept the challenges you will bump into in pursuit of your goals. Meditating on your goals, watching them play out over and over again, will put your mental defenses in action so you can ultimately be positive, happy, and a victor.

HIGH-KNEE WALL HIKE

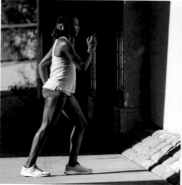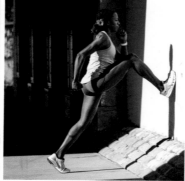

From a staggered stance swing your back leg forward to touch down on the wall as close to hip-height as possible. Swing back to reload, pumping your arms in opposition with your legs. Work both sides.

 ## JACK SQUAT

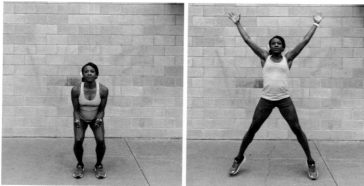

Start from a squat, arms tucked; then pop up and out into the jack position, legs and arms out. Spring from squat to jack and back without pausing.

STEP-UP

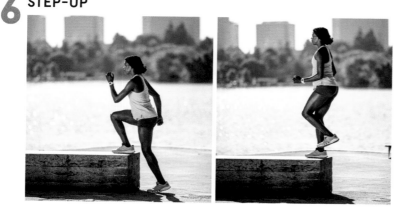

Step one foot onto the bench. Push through that leg to bring your back leg up and drive your knee toward your chest. Pump your arms opposite your legs. Lower back down with control. Work both sides.

TOTAL-BODY MUSCLE ENDURANCE

Get ready to build muscle stamina, better running form, and improved staying power. By focusing on perceived exertion, or how hard you feel like your muscles are working, it ensures that you hit that burn-so-good point that's required for muscle growth.

▶ **Do each exercise until you reach an RPE of 8 to 9. You should almost hit "failure," that moment when your muscles give out. Use a 3:1:1 tempo, resting 15 seconds between moves. Rest for 1 minute between rounds if performing them back-to-back. Complete a total of 3 rounds throughout the day.**

1 WALL SIT ▶ Hold 30–40 seconds for each set.

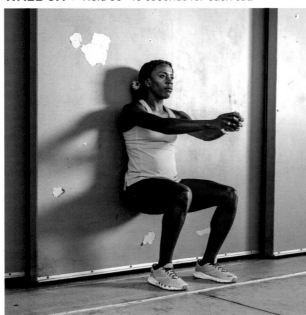

Using a wall for support, sink into a seated position where your quads are parallel with the ground. And hold.

2 PUSH-UP WITH LEG LIFT

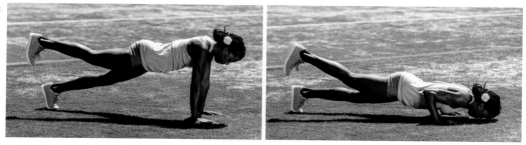

From a high-plank position, raise one leg and lower your body down, elbows tucked in, and back up. Alternate sides.

« PUSH-UP

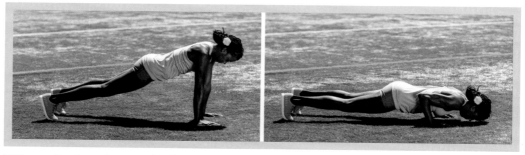

With your hands under your shoulders, squeeze your back, abs, and glutes to hold your body in a straight line. Lower your body to the ground, keeping your elbows tucked; then press back up.

3 SINGLE-LEG SQUAT

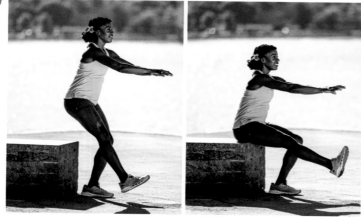

Stand on one leg and sit back until your butt lightly touches the bench. Press through the standing leg to return to standing. Extend your arms in front for balance as you squat down, slow and controlled. Work both sides. » Lower without a raised surface behind you.

REAR-FOOT-ELEVATED SPLIT SQUAT

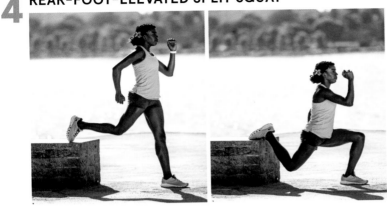

Stand on one leg and position your opposite foot behind you on a bench. Lower your hips down into a squat and drive through your heel to come back up. Work both sides.

5

BENT-OVER BAND ROW

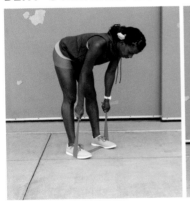
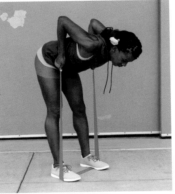

Anchor the middle of the band under both feet and hinge forward at the hips. Keeping your elbows tucked, pull the band up toward your chest. Return to the start position, slow and controlled.

DUCK WALK

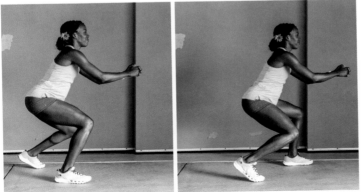

Walk forward in a squat stance, heel first, pushing through the toe. Walk backward reversing the foot motion, rolling toe to heel.

FLEXIBILITY + MOBILITY

Warning: This workout is going to feel great, especially if you're tired, achy, or stiff. It will help you move in new, healthier ways, and reduce the risk of running (or everyday life) injury.

▶ Perform 2 rounds of each circuit, completing 12 to 16 reps of each mobility exercise. Rest for 15 seconds between circuits if performing them back-to-back. Make sure to check off each circuit by the end of the day.

CIRCUIT 1

DONKEY WHIP

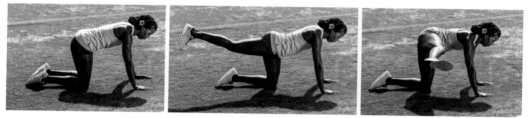

Extend one leg straight behind you; then whip it up to the side and back in a fluid, controlled motion. Engage your core and glute on the supporting side. Work both sides.

HIP CIRCLES

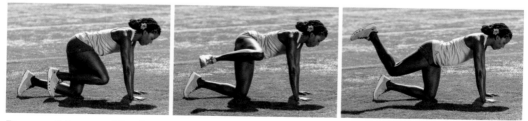

From an all-fours position, keep your core engaged as you lift your knee first out to the side, then around and behind you, and then forward to start another circle. Halfway through your reps, reverse direction. Work the other side.

HIP SWITCH

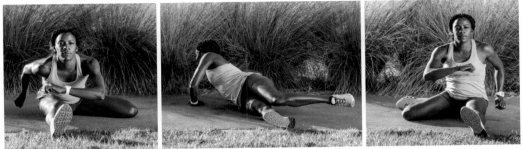

Sit with one leg extended and your other leg bent at a 90-degree angle behind you. Lean forward with the opposite arm leading the stretch. Now swing your back leg around and roll laterally into a stretch on the opposite side. Find your rhythm, moving dynamically from side to side.

CIRCUIT 2

WALL SLIDE

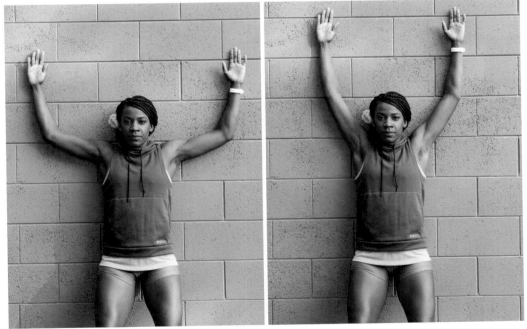

Stand with your butt, shoulders, elbows, and hands against the wall. Extend your arms up the wall, trying to limit the arch in your low back; then lower your body back down the wall.

FORWARD LEG SWING

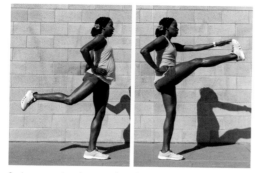

Swing one leg forward and back. Hold a wall for stability if needed. Repeat on the other side.

SIDEWAYS LEG SWING

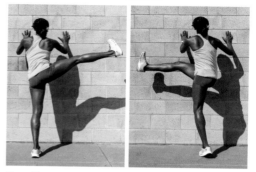

Face the wall and swing one leg from side to side. Work the other side.

HURDLE WALK-OVERS

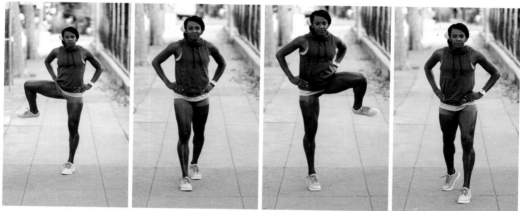

Lift one leg up and out to the side as if you were stepping over a hurdle and moving forward; continue alternating legs.

SIDE HURDLE

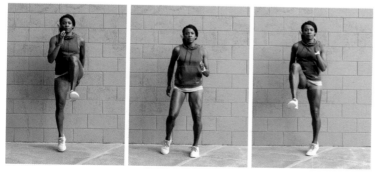

Lift one leg up and step out to the side as if you are stepping over a hurdle, and follow with the trailing leg coming up and over the hurdle. Keep it going, and halfway through the reps, switch direction.

▶ Hold each stretch for 5 seconds, take a breath, and see if you can stretch a little farther. Do this 5–6 times, then repeat on the other side.

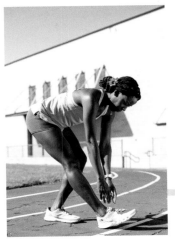

STANDING HAMSTRING STRETCH

Extend one leg just out in front of you and let the knee of the opposite leg bend as you reach forward. Try to keep your back flat.

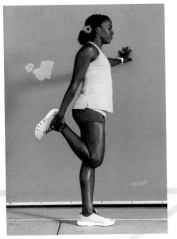

STANDING QUAD STRETCH

Using a wall for support, stand on one leg and pull the opposite heel to your glute. Press forward through your stretched side to keep your hips and knees square.

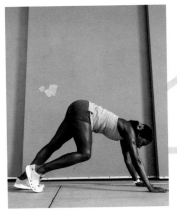

DOWNWARD DOG CALF STRETCH

Push your palms and heels into the ground, bending one knee at a time as you push the opposite heel to the ground to stretch that calf.

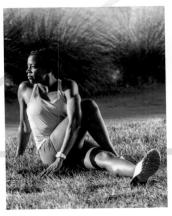

SEATED SPINAL ROTATION

With legs extended, cross one leg over the other and twist in the opposite direction, using your arm to push your knee in toward your chest.

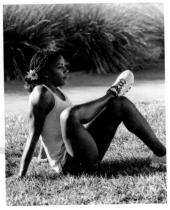

SEATED GLUTE STRETCH

With knees bent, cross one leg over the other to get into a figure-4 position. Gently move closer to your stationary foot to intensify the stretch.

PLYOMETRIC RUNNING DRILLS

These explosive plyo moves are all about improving power and nailing your running form and mechanics. Get ready to spring off the start line and sprint toward the finish line with a new level of oomph!

WARM-UP

▶ Complete an easy 10-minute jog, trying to maintain a consistent pace (RPE 3 to 4) throughout.

▶ Do each exercise for 30 seconds, "resting" for 30 seconds between exercises by performing High Knees. Rest for 1 minute between rounds if performing them back-to-back. Complete a total of 5 rounds throughout the day.

HIGH KNEES

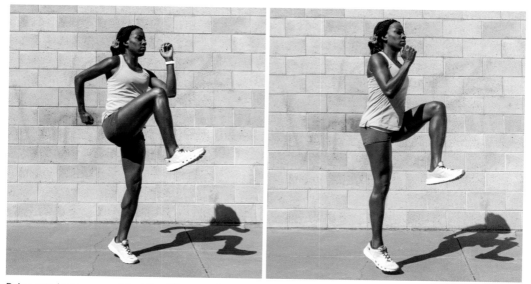

Drive one knee up, and feel the lift as you hop-skip up to the ball of your foot; alternate sides. Drive your arms in a tight stride, opposite your legs.

SPLIT SQUAT JUMP

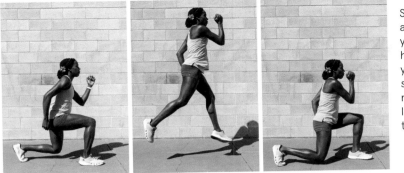

Start in a split stance and pop up. Switch your stance as you hit the height of your jump and land soft. Get your arms moving opposite your legs so you can tap that momentum.

SKATER JUMP

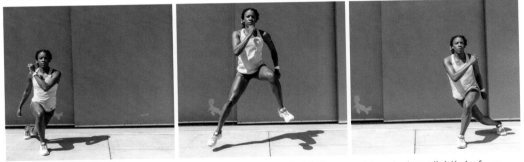

Jump from side to side. As you land, swing the inside leg behind you and touch down lightly before bounding back to the other side.

X JUMP

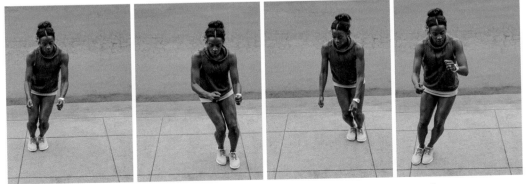

Keep your feet together as you jump from corner to corner, hitting all four corners of a square—diagonally forward, back, diagonally forward, then back to the first corner. Switch directions halfway through the rep count.

CORE STRENGTH

Your core is going to be wiped after this! Resist the urge to skip your rest intervals. You're going to need that rest to perform effective, and safe, reps.

▶ **Perform 3 to 4 rounds of each circuit, completing 12 to 16 reps of each exercise and resting for 30 seconds between rounds. Rest for 1 minute between circuits if performing them back-to-back. Check off both circuits by the end of the day.**

CIRCUIT 1

1 LATERAL BEAR CRAWL

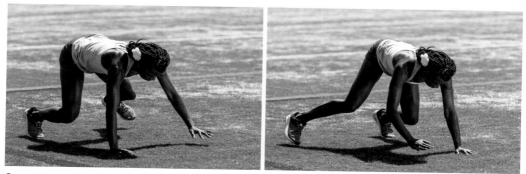

Come to your hands and the balls of your feet, and step to the side with one hand and the adjacent foot; then follow with the opposing hand and foot. Keep your core engaged, back flat, and butt down. Halfway through the reps, move back in the opposite direction.

2 TWISTING SUPERWOMAN

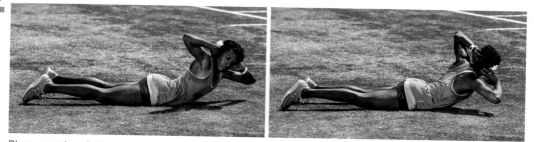

Place your hands behind your head and engage your trunk muscles to lift and twist your torso from side to side with control. Back off the lift slightly if you feel the load in your low back.

REVERSE PLANK WITH LATERAL EXTENSION

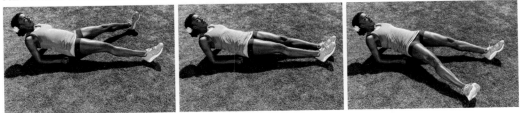

Lean back on your elbows and lift your body into plank position. Engage your core as you lift one leg out and in. Alternate sides.

HEEL TOUCH

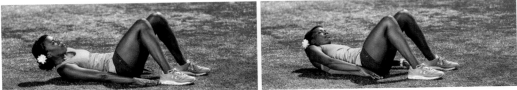

Engage your core just enough to lift your shoulders off the ground, and hold that position as you reach for your heel. Alternate side to side.

CIRCUIT 2

V-UP

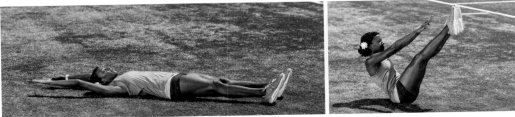

Extend your arms overhead and engage your core as you lift your legs and reach up and forward, toward your feet. Come back down with control. Keep your arms, legs, and back as straight as possible.

« BICYCLE CRUNCH

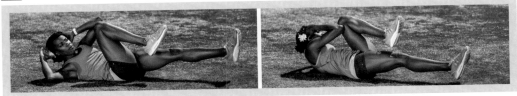

Engage your core as you pull your elbow and the opposite knee toward each other, alternating side to side.

2 HIP LIFT

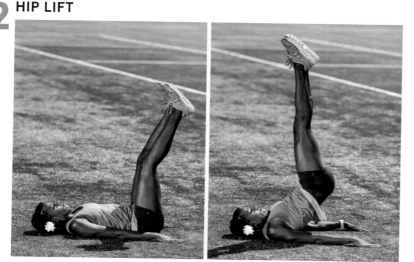

Use your core to push your hips and reach your feet upward. Come back down with control.

3 LYING SCISSOR KICK

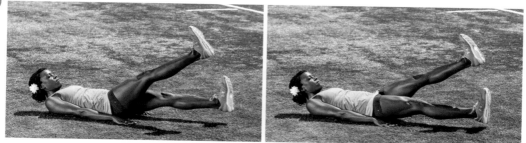

Engage your core holding your shoulders and legs just off the ground as you "scissor" your legs up, then back down. Keep your low back flat on the ground.

4 DEAD BUG

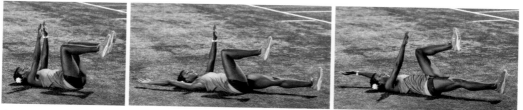

Get set with your low back flat on the ground, arms extended up, knees bent. Now move your opposing arm and leg to reach long while you move the opposite hand toward your knee. Keep alternating the movement, slow and controlled.

Challenge 7

PUT SETBACKS IN THE REARVIEW MIRROR

You may have heard the saying, "Every setback is a setup for a comeback." Well, there's a reason clichés are cliché: They are usually true. But here's the thing: Nothing gets done if you don't take action.

Whether you're coming back from injury, illness, pregnancy, or just an extended break from exercise, this challenge will get you in the right headspace to remember you are in charge of your health and fitness. You can overcome any barrier to your success with a little help and a lot of hard work.

The first step to getting back on the saddle is getting up! So get up, saddle up, and get ready to ride this four-week routine. Throughout it, you'll focus on getting back into a habit and hitting all areas of fitness, with a big emphasis on mobility, joint health, and both prehabilitation and rehabilitation work.

Like Coach Sandoval (my track and field coach at UC Berkeley) always says, "It's time to take care of the small things so that the big things will take care of themselves!"

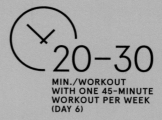

20–30

MIN./WORKOUT
WITH ONE 45-MINUTE
WORKOUT PER WEEK
(DAY 6)

6 days per week for *4 weeks*

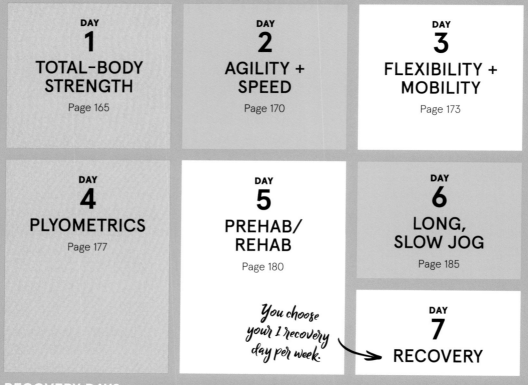

DAY
1
TOTAL-BODY
STRENGTH

Page 165

DAY
2
AGILITY +
SPEED

Page 170

DAY
3
FLEXIBILITY +
MOBILITY

Page 173

DAY
4
PLYOMETRICS

Page 177

DAY
5
PREHAB/
REHAB

Page 180

DAY
6
LONG,
SLOW JOG

Page 185

You choose your 1 recovery day per week.

DAY
7
RECOVERY

RECOVERY DAYS If you do want to get a little recovery work in, check out the **Foam Rolling** and **Mobility** routines in the Appendix (p. 270).

EQUIPMENT Running shoes ▪ dumbbells ▪ 2 resistance bands (1 short, 1 long) ▪ rope ▪ foam roller

TOTAL-BODY STRENGTH

Strengthen every muscle with this superset-based routine. During each superset, you'll focus on perceived exertion, or how hard it feels like your muscles are working. This ensures that you're triggering true change.

▶ **Perform each exercise in the superset to fatigue, rest for 15 seconds, and then repeat for 3 rounds. Rest for 45 to 60 seconds between supersets.**

1 SUMO SQUAT WITH PRESS

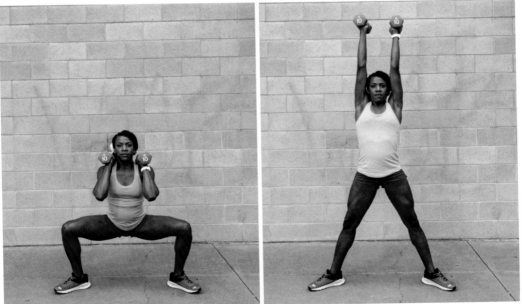

Get into a wide sumo stance, toes pointed outward and weights in front of your shoulders. Squat down and drive through your heels, pressing the weights overhead. Keep your core engaged—you shouldn't feel the load in your low back.

DEADLIFT TO BENT-OVER ROW

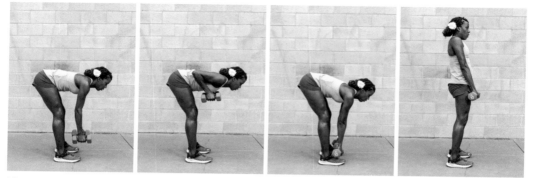

Hinge at the hips and lower the weights close to your body, until your back is parallel with the ground. Turn your palms inward. Pinch your shoulder blades together as you "row," pulling the weights up to your torso (with elbows tucked); then lower back down. Now push your ribs forward to return to standing.

2 SIDE LUNGE, WITH WEIGHTS

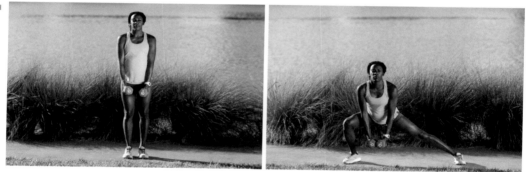

Step out to one side into a lunge; then push off back to start. Work both sides.

LATERAL BEAR CRAWL

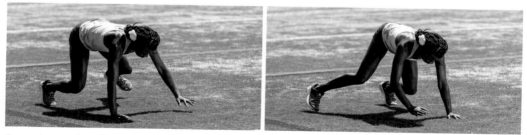

Come to your hands and the balls of your feet, and step to the side with one hand and the adjacent foot; then follow with the opposing hand and foot. Keep your core engaged, back flat, and butt down. Halfway through the reps, move back in the opposite direction.

3 SINGLE-LEG SQUAT

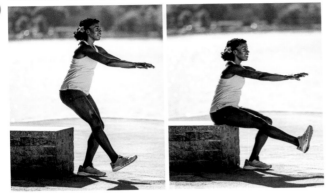

Stand on one leg and sit back until your butt lightly touches the bench. Press through the standing leg to return to standing. Extend your arms in front for balance as you squat down, slow and controlled. Work both sides.

INCLINE PUSH-UP, LEG EXTENDED

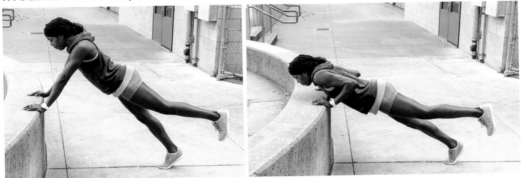

Start in push-up position, with one leg lifted, positioning your hands on a wall or high step. Keeping your body in a straight line, lower your body toward your hands, keeping your elbows tucked; then return to start. Work both sides.

» PUSH-UP WITH LEG LIFT

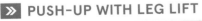

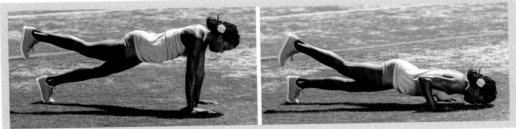

From a high-plank position, raise one leg and lower your body down, elbows tucked in, and back up. Alternate sides.

4 WEIGHTED REVERSE LUNGE TO KNEE DRIVE

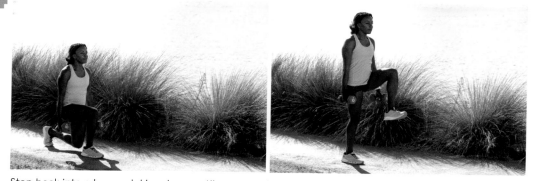

Step back into a lunge, sinking down until your quad is parallel with the ground. Then push off your back foot and bring your knee high before stepping back into a lunge again. Do all of the reps on one side, then switch. Let your legs do the work.

OVERHEAD TRICEPS EXTENSION

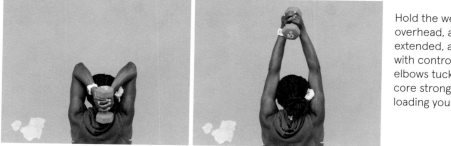

Hold the weight overhead, arms extended, and lower it with control. Keep your elbows tucked and your core strong to avoid loading your low back.

Mental toughness

Your mind is the greatest muscle you'll flex in your fitness pursuit. Not everything comes easy or naturally, you have to work at it . . . and then when you are physically exhausted, it's time to home in on mind over matter. Pushing through mental blocks inevitably makes you tougher and stronger, so give your mind some gym work too. Instill positive thoughts and words both in your workouts and throughout your day, acknowledge small victories as they happen, and remember that hard is just part of the journey.

The adage rings true: Whether you think you can or you think you can't, you're right. When that inner voice tells you that you can't, it's time to face the mirror and rally up some affirmation—just like you would do for a friend. Give yourself mantras to put that inner voice in check and win yourself over to the idea that yes, you can. Affirmations allow you to flex your mental muscle and become the mental warrior that you were destined to be.

5 SIDE PLANK, THREAD THE NEEDLE

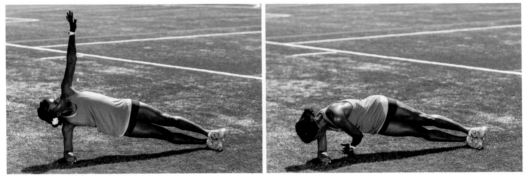

Hold a side plank. Reach your opposite arm up high, then under your torso. Track your hand with your eyes as you continue the movement. Work both sides.

STANDING CALF RAISE

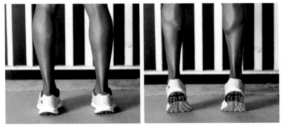

Push through the balls of your feet to raise your heels as high as possible; then lower back down with control. Hold on to a stationary object for balance if needed.

» ELEVATED SINGLE-LEG CALF RAISE

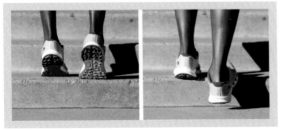

Use a step to work one calf at a time in a fuller range of motion. Stand on a step, keeping all of your weight on one working leg. The other foot is just there for balance. Lower your heel as far as possible with control; then push through the ball of that foot to raise your heel as high as possible. Work both sides.

WEEKLY PROGRESSIONS
Week 2: Use a 2:1:1 tempo.
Week 3: Use a 3:1:1 tempo.
Week 4: Use a 4:1:1 tempo.
See p. 14 Count Your Tempo

AGILITY + SPEED

For better athleticism, we'll train your reaction time, ability to change directions, and speed with fun, engaging drills.

WARM-UP

Complete an easy 5-minute walk or jog, trying to maintain a consistent pace (RPE 3 to 4) throughout.

AGILITY DRILLS

▶ Perform 30 seconds of each exercise, resting for 30 seconds between each one. Rest for 1 minute; then repeat the entire circuit for a total of 2 to 3 rounds.

1 LATERAL LADDER

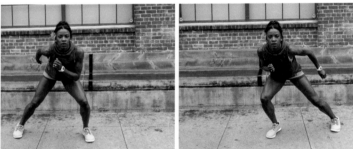

Get in a wide athletic stance and shuffle your feet from side to side, keeping your weight over the inside foot. Pump your arms for momentum and move as quickly as possible. Fast feet!

2 FORWARD LADDER SHUFFLE

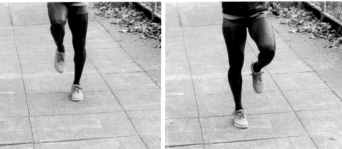

Keeping your feet under your body, spring forward onto one leg, then the other. Move forward with each step as if you're stepping between the rungs of an agility ladder. Pump your arms opposite your fast feet!

3 SIDE-TO-SIDE HOP-OVER

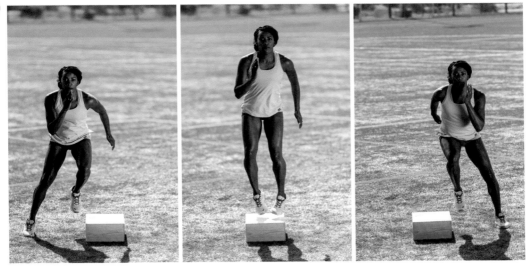

Move from side to side over the top of a step or stationary object, with a quick stutter-step at the top or midpoint. Get your arms pumping opposite your legs for added momentum.

4 X JUMP

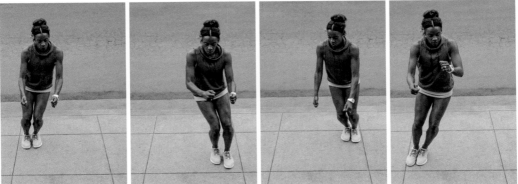

Keep your feet together as you jump from corner to corner, hitting all four corners of a square—diagonally forward, back, diagonally forward, then back to the first corner. Switch directions halfway through the rep count.

5 SIDE HURDLE

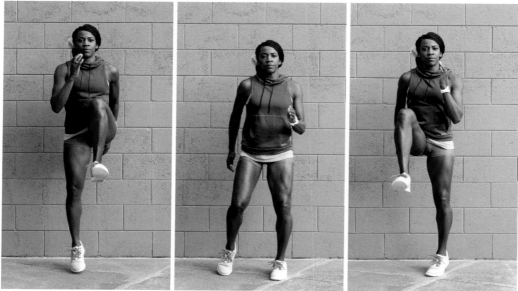

Lift one leg up and step out to the side as if you are stepping over a hurdle, and follow with the trailing leg coming up and over the hurdle. Keep it going, and halfway through the reps, switch direction.

RUN

SPEEDWORK   **4 × 15-second max sprints (RPE 9 to 10)**

Run with concentrated, exaggerated, fluid form. Pump your arms and legs. Between each sprint, slow to a fast walk or slow jog until your heart rate has come down; then hit it again!

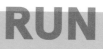

WEEKLY PROGRESSIONS
Week 2: Perform 5 sprints.
Week 3: Perform 6 sprints.
Week 4: Perform 7 sprints.

FLEXIBILITY + MOBILITY

Each move will feel like a cross between a strength exercise and a stretch to relieve tension; help you move in new, healthier ways; and reduce your risk of running (or everyday life) injury.

▶ **Perform each exercise in the superset for 30 seconds back-to-back, and repeat for 3 rounds. Rest for 15 seconds between supersets.**

1 DONKEY KICK TO FIRE HYDRANT

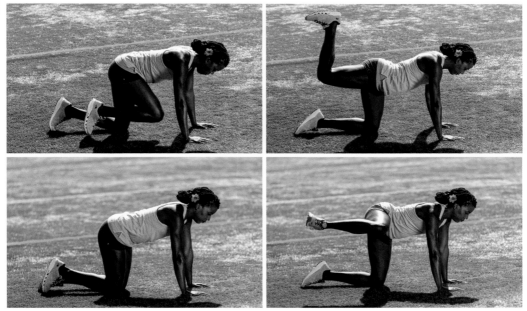

Get on all fours, and engage your glutes to raise your foot up behind you and lower it back down with control. Then lift the same leg out laterally and lower with control. Use your core to keep your back flat and feel the glutes burn, even on the stationary leg. Work both sides.

STRAIGHT-LEG HIP CIRCLES

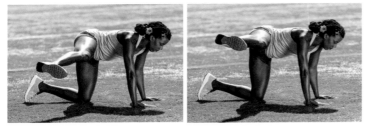

Engage your glutes to raise one leg straight out to your side. In one fluid motion, make a circle with your foot. Halfway through your reps, reverse direction. Work the other side.

« HIP CIRCLES

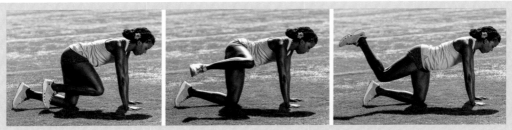

From an all-fours position, keep your core engaged as you lift your knee first out to the side, then around and behind you, and then forward to start another circle. Halfway through your reps, reverse direction. Work the other side.

2 FORWARD LEG SWING

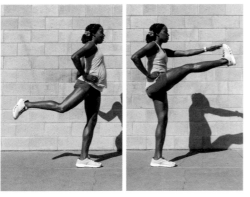

Swing one leg forward and back. Hold a wall for stability if needed. Repeat on the other side.

SIDEWAYS LEG SWING

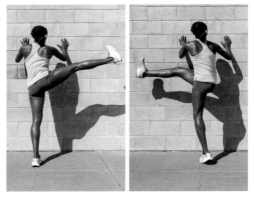

Face the wall and swing one leg from side to side. Work the other side.

3 COBRA SUPERWOMAN TO LOW SUPERWOMAN

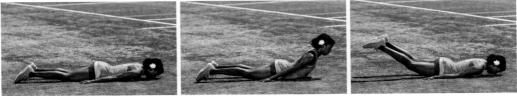

Start with your arms at your sides, palms down, and engage your trunk muscles to lift and lower your torso with control. Use your glutes to lift and lower your legs with control. Back off the lift slightly if you feel the load in your low back.

TWISTING MOUNTAIN CLIMBER

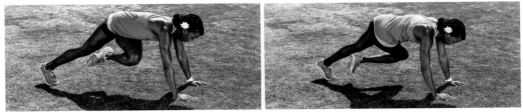

From high-plank position, bring your knee in toward the opposite elbow; alternate from side to side.

4 HIP SWITCH

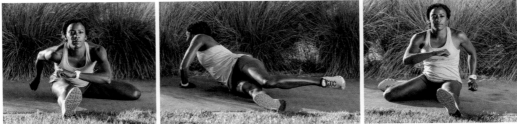

Sit with one leg extended and your other leg bent at a 90-degree angle behind you. Lean forward with the opposite arm leading the stretch. Now swing your back leg around and roll laterally into a stretch on the opposite side. Find your rhythm, moving dynamically from side to side.

SEATED SPINAL ROTATION

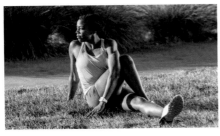

With legs extended, cross one leg over the other and twist in the opposite direction, using your arm to push your knee in toward your chest. Stretch both sides.

▶ Stretch for 5–10 seconds and release. Repeat, maybe taking it a little farther as you exhale. After a few sets, work the other side.

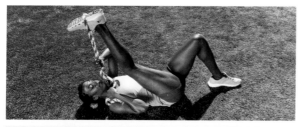

HAMSTRING ROPE STRETCH

Keeping your foot flexed, pull your leg toward your chest. Gently straighten your knee to deepen the stretch.

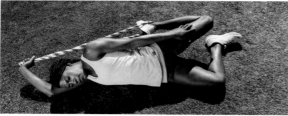

QUAD ROPE STRETCH

Lying on your side, pull your foot toward your butt, keeping it flexed. Let your knee travel behind your hips.

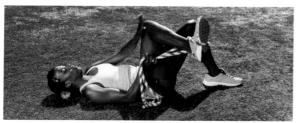

ABDUCTOR ROPE STRETCH

Use the rope to gently pull your foot out to one side, using your hand to keep your knee aligned with your hip.

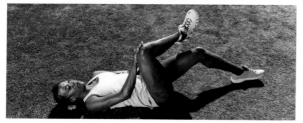

ADDUCTOR ROPE STRETCH

Use the rope to gently pull one foot in toward your torso, using your hand to keep your knee aligned with your hip.

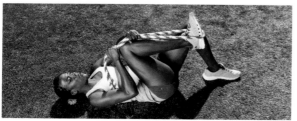

GLUTE ROPE STRETCH

Bring one knee in toward your chest, using the rope to deepen the stretch.

PLYOMETRICS

All of the muscles in your body have specialized elastic components, which act similarly to rubber bands or springs. These plyo exercises will train those components, making you more efficient, responsive, and powerful.

WARM-UP

▶ Complete an easy 10-minute jog, trying to maintain a consistent pace (RPE 3 to 4) throughout.

CIRCUIT 1

▶ Do each exercise for 30 seconds, resting 30 seconds between moves. (Take your time and don't worry about how many reps you do.) Repeat for a total of 4 rounds, resting for 1 minute between rounds.

1 ROLY-POLY POWER JUMP

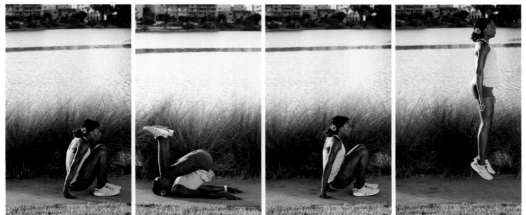

Start in a standing position, sit down, roll backward bringing your knees to chest; then quickly roll up onto your feet and power up into a jump.

2 SKATER JUMP

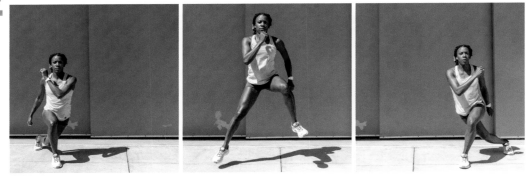

Jump from side to side. As you land, swing the inside leg behind you and touch down lightly before bounding back to the other side.

3 HIGH KNEES

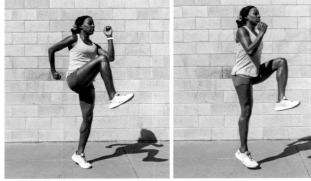

Drive one knee up, and feel the lift as you hop-skip up to the ball of your foot; alternate sides. Drive your arms in a tight stride, opposite your legs.

4 SPLIT SQUAT JUMP

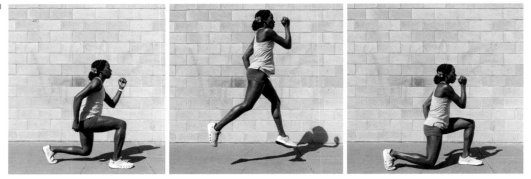

Start in a split stance and pop up. Switch your stance as you hit the height of your jump and land soft. Get your arms moving opposite your legs so you can tap that momentum.

5 SINGLE-LEG POWER-UP

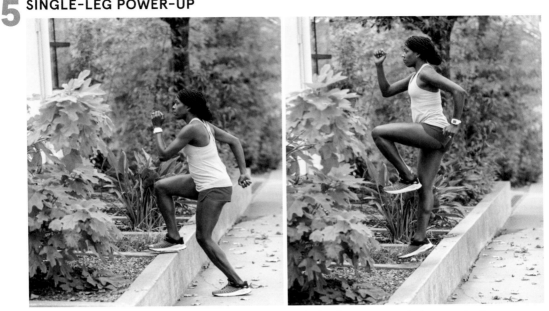

Start with one foot up on a bench or step. Drive through that leg as you explode up and raise your opposite knee toward your chest; then land soft and step back down. Keep a steady rhythm, moving your arms opposite your legs to create momentum. Work both sides.

6 FORWARD BOUND

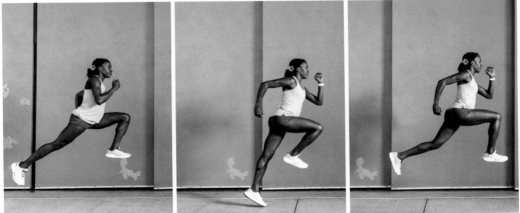

Bound forward, driving off of each foot, and landing soft.

PREHAB/REHAB

To truly put setbacks (especially injuries!) in the rearview mirror, it's important to integrate prehabilitation and rehabilitation exercises into your routine. These moves strengthen commonly undertrained muscles to improve recovery, muscle balance, and form, and to prevent aches and pains down the road.

▶ **Perform 3 rounds of each circuit, performing each exercise for 30 seconds and resting for 30 seconds between rounds. Rest for 1 minute between circuits.**

CIRCUIT 1

GLUTE ROLL

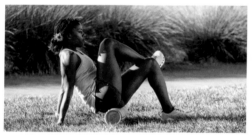

Cross one leg into a figure-4 position and roll out the glute of the stationary leg with a foam roller. Switch sides.

CALF ROLL

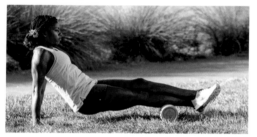

Roll out your calf muscle, using your opposite leg to go a little deeper. Switch sides.

UPPER-BACK ROLL

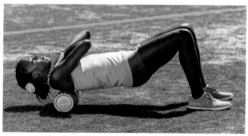

Position a foam roller under your shoulders and lift your hips. Move your feet to shift the roller up and down your back.

HIP FLEXOR ROLL

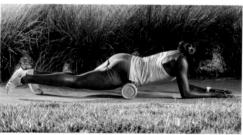

Stabilize yourself with one foot and gently roll out your hip flexor on the opposite leg. Work the other side.

1 LATERAL BAND WALK

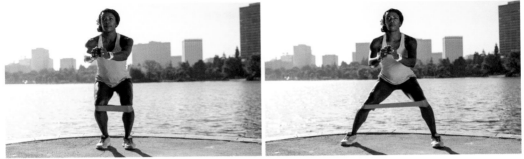

Place the band just below your knees. From a half-squat stance, step one foot out to the side and follow with the opposite foot, keeping the band taut at all times. Return in the opposite direction to work the other side.

2 BAND WALK

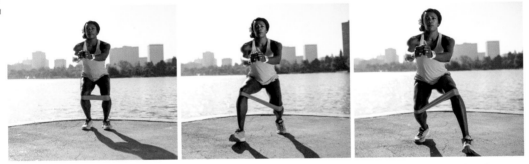

Stand with your feet shoulder-width apart and walk forward, heel-to-toe, keeping the band taut. Halfway through the reps walk backward, toe-to-heel.

3 DUCK WALK

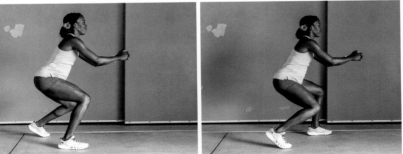

Walk forward in a squat stance, heel first, pushing through the toe. Walk backward, reversing the foot motion, rolling toe to heel.

BAND PULL-APART

1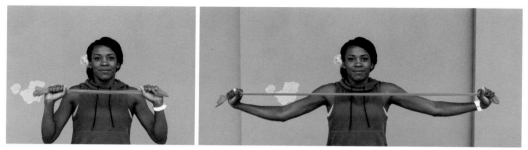

Hold the band palms out, with hands just outside of shoulder-width. Engage your core and pull until your arms (and the band) are fully extended.

LAWNMOWER RESISTANCE BAND ROW

2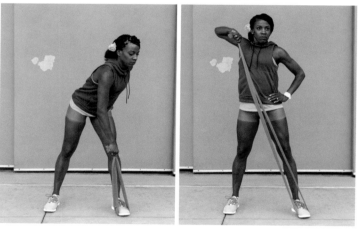

Anchor the band under one foot and hold it in the opposite hand. Pull the band up toward your shoulder, keeping your core engaged and elbow high. Return to the start position, slow and controlled. Work both sides.

ELEVATED SINGLE-LEG CALF RAISE

3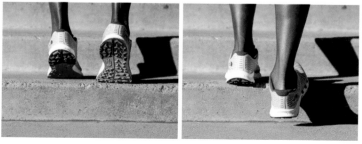

Stand on a step, keeping all of your weight on one working leg. The other foot is just there for balance. Lower your heel as far as possible with control; then push through the ball of that foot to raise your heel as high as possible. Work both sides.

4 SINGLE-LEG DEADLIFT TO KNEE DRIVE

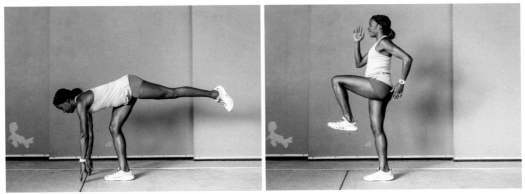

Balance on one leg, extending the opposite leg straight behind you, and tip forward. Keep your back flat and pendulum-swing your leg back up to a high-knee stance. Work both sides.

CIRCUIT 4

1 DEAD BUG

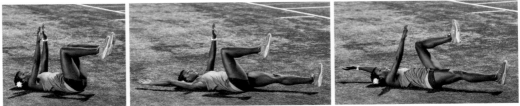

Get set with your low back flat on the ground, arms extended up, knees bent. Now move your opposing arm and leg to reach long while you move the opposite hand toward your knee. Keep alternating the movement, slow and controlled.

2 SIDE PLANK, THREAD THE NEEDLE

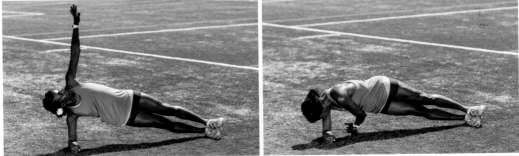

Hold a side plank. Reach your opposite arm up high, then under your torso. Track your hand with your eyes as you continue the movement. Work both sides.

3 I, Y, AND T RAISES

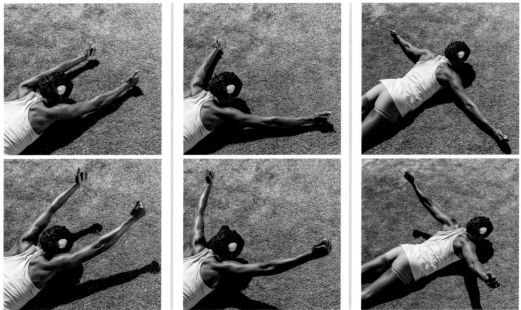

Lie down and squeeze your shoulder blades together to raise and lower your arms overhead in an "I" position, slow and controlled. Move from your shoulders, with your thumbs leading the way. Repeat to get in your Y and T raises.

4 HAMSTRING CURL

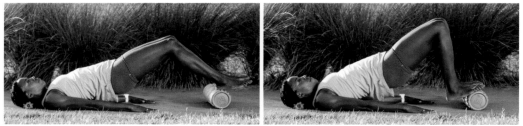

Lie on your back with the foam roller under your heels. Lift your hips up and pull your heels in until the roller reaches your toes. Continue rolling out and in.

LONG, SLOW JOG

Today is all about building muscular and aerobic endurance. We aren't pushing the pace, aiming for high-intensity work, or jacking our heart rate to a high degree.

WARM-UP

▶ Complete an easy 5-minute run, trying to maintain a consistent pace (RPE 3 to 4) throughout.

ACTIVATION DRILLS

▶ Do 6 reps of exercises 1–3, resting 15 seconds between each exercise. Repeat for a total of 2 rounds.

1 DONKEY WHIP

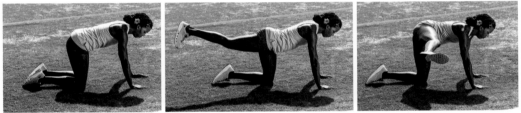

Extend one leg straight behind you; then whip it up to the side and back in a fluid, controlled motion. Engage your core and glute on the supporting side. Work both sides.

2 HEEL TOUCH

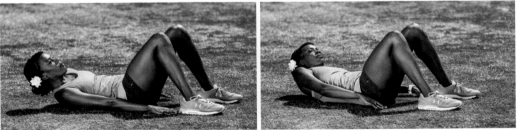

Engage your core just enough to lift your shoulders off the ground, and hold that position as you reach for your heel. Alternate side to side.

3 SIDE LUNGE TO KNEE DRIVE

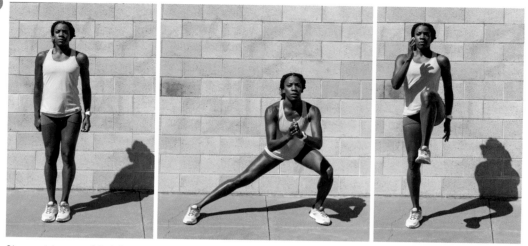

Step out to one side into a squat; then push up into a sprinter position, knee high. Work both sides.

▶ Do 6 reps of Exercises 4–5, resting 15 seconds between each exercise. Repeat for a total of 2 rounds.

4 LATERAL BAND WALK

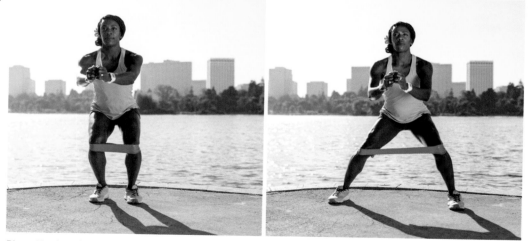

Place the band just below your knees. From a half-squat stance, step one foot out to the side and follow with the opposite foot, keeping the band taut at all times. Return in the opposite direction to work the other side.

5 BAND WALK

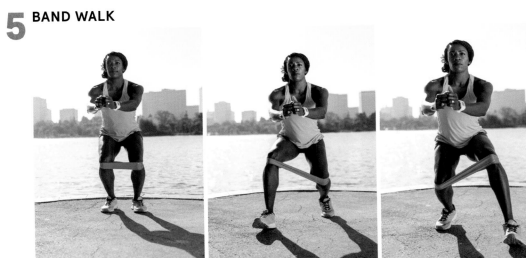

Stand with your feet shoulder-width apart and walk forward, heel-to-toe, keeping the band taut. Halfway through the reps walk backward, toe-to-heel.

RUN

LONG, SLOW JOG Run or jog for 30 minutes, focusing on keeping a nice, easy pace (RPE 4 to 5) that would allow you to carry on a conversation with a workout buddy or sing along with whatever is playing on your headphones.

WEEKLY PROGRESSIONS
You may be able to shave some time off your pace from week to week, but focus on maintaining a nice, easy pace and not turning this run into a race.

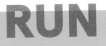

▶ Hold each stretch for 5 seconds, take a breath, and see if you can stretch a little farther. Do this 5–6 times, then repeat on the other side.

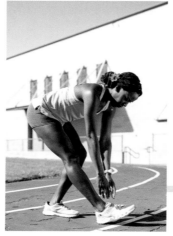

STANDING HAMSTRING STRETCH

Extend one leg just out in front of you and let the knee of the opposite leg bend as you reach forward. Try to keep your back flat.

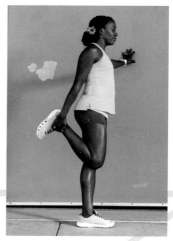

STANDING QUAD STRETCH

Using a wall for support, stand on one leg and pull the opposite heel to your glute. Press forward through your stretched side to keep your hips and knees square.

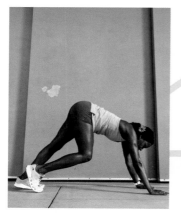

DOWNWARD DOG CALF STRETCH

Push your palms and heels into the ground, bending one knee at a time as you push the opposite heel to the ground to stretch that calf.

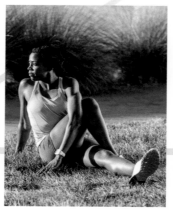

SEATED SPINAL ROTATION

With legs extended, cross one leg over the other and twist in the opposite direction, using your arm to push your knee in toward your chest.

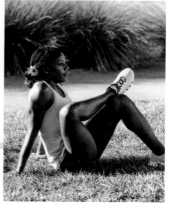

SEATED GLUTE STRETCH

With knees bent, cross one leg over the other to get into a figure-4 position. Gently move closer to your stationary foot to intensify the stretch.

Challenge 8

PUSH YOUR LIMITS

Inside, we all have that tiny voice: the one that tells us that we can't. It tells us to slow down or we won't make it. It tells us that it's hard enough, and we can stop right there. No need to work harder or go farther.

That little voice speaks up hundreds of times before we ever truly push our bodies to their limits. This challenge will prove just that, pushing you to achieve what that little voice has always said is impossible. Each week, you'll perform six challenging, limit-testing workouts.

You'll run harder, faster, and longer than you have in any of your previous challenges. You'll lift more weight, jump higher, churn out more reps, and hit every exercise with focus, intention, and belief in yourself.

I believe in you!

Redefining limits

FLOWER POWER

Fear is totally normal and necessary for survival. As I see it, bravery is not the absence of fear, but the ability to take flight in its presence. What are you afraid of—failing? With every challenge that you take on, you are redefining your limits and discovering what you are capable of. Ladders exist so that when heights seem too high, out of our reach, we can find a way to make it happen. Grab a ladder and climb past that nagging question of "What if?" and the limits that you currently know. Keep going.

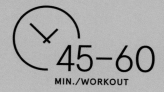

45–60
MIN./WORKOUT

6 days per week for *5 weeks*

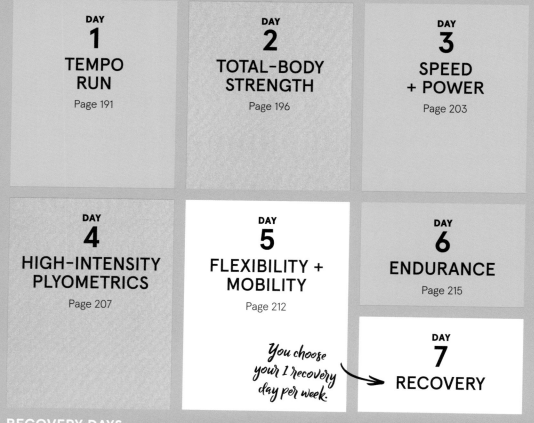

DAY
1
TEMPO
RUN
Page 191

DAY
2
TOTAL-BODY
STRENGTH
Page 196

DAY
3
SPEED
+ POWER
Page 203

DAY
4
HIGH-INTENSITY
PLYOMETRICS
Page 207

DAY
5
FLEXIBILITY +
MOBILITY
Page 212

DAY
6
ENDURANCE
Page 215

You choose your 1 recovery day per week.

DAY
7
RECOVERY

RECOVERY DAYS If you do want to get a little recovery work in, check out the **Foam Rolling** and **Mobility** routines in the Appendix (p. 270).

EQUIPMENT Running shoes ▪ dumbbells ▪ 2 resistance bands (1 short, 1 long) ▪ medicine ball ▪ kettlebell ▪ rope ▪ foam rollers

TEMPO RUN

Train your body to run faster and longer without fatiguing by increasing the amount of work your aerobic system can handle.

WARM-UP

▶ Complete an easy 10-minute jog, trying to maintain a consistent pace (RPE 3 to 4) throughout.

ACTIVATION DRILLS

▶ Complete each superset by doing 6 to 8 reps of each exercise back-to-back without rest. Repeat for a total of 2 rounds, resting for 15 seconds between each round and superset.

1 **FORWARD LEG SWING**

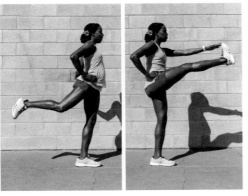

Swing one leg forward and back. Hold a wall for stability if needed. Repeat on the other side.

SIDEWAYS LEG SWING

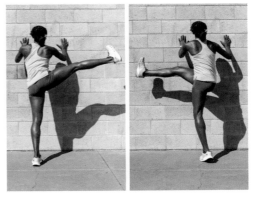

Face the wall and swing one leg from side to side. Work the other side.

2 BAND WALK

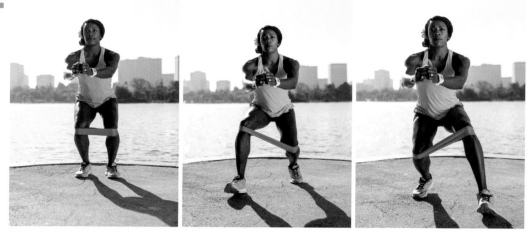

Place the band at or just above your knees. Start from a half-squat stance with your feet shoulder-width apart and walk forward, heel-to-toe, keeping the band taut. Halfway through the reps walk backward, toe-to-heel.

LATERAL BAND WALK

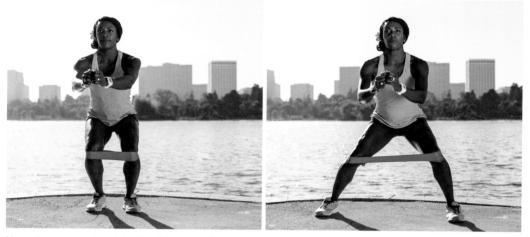

Now step one foot out to the side and follow with the opposite foot, keeping the band taut. Return in the opposite direction to work the other side.

3 SINGLE-LEG POWER-UP

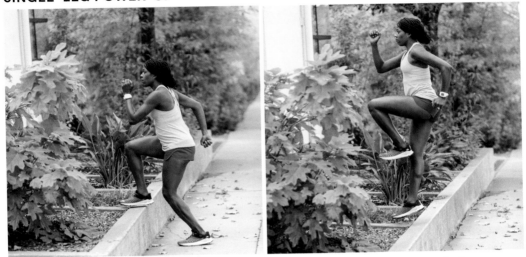

Start with one foot up on a bench or step. Drive through that leg as you explode up and raise your opposite knee toward your chest; then land soft and step back down. Keep a steady rhythm, moving your arms opposite your legs to create momentum. Work both sides.

INCHWORM WITH PUSH-UP

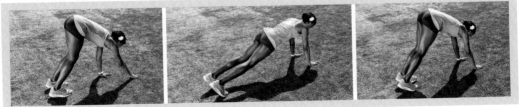

Get into a forward fold and walk your hands out into a high plank. Do a push-up. Then walk your feet in until you are in a forward fold again. And keep on going.

« INCHWORM

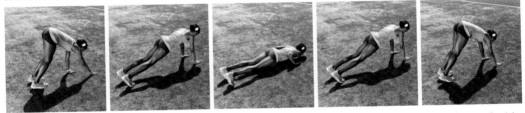

Get into a forward fold and walk your hands out into a high plank. Then walk your feet in until you are in a forward fold again. And keep on going.

4 SKATER JUMP

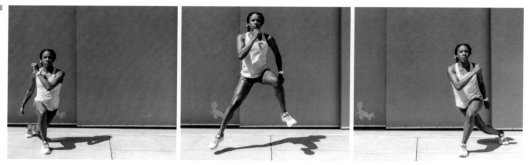

Jump from side to side. As you land, swing the inside leg behind you and touch down lightly before bounding back to the other side.

BAND PULL-APART

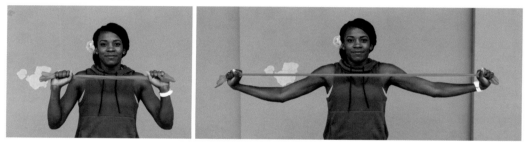

Hold the band palms out, with hands just outside of shoulder-width. Engage your core and pull until your arms (and the band) are fully extended.

RUN

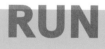

TEMPO **Run for 30 minutes (RPE 5 to 6).**

Try to maintain a challenging but doable pace that you feel you could keep up for an extra 10 more minutes if you needed. If you add about 60 seconds to your mile time trial pace, this is likely close to your ideal tempo pace. Not sure what your mile pace is? Just pay attention to how it feels.

WEEKLY PROGRESSIONS
Try to shave a few seconds off your pace each week. Pay attention to your breathing and form to increase your speed without increasing how hard you feel you're working.

▶ Hold each stretch for 5 seconds, take a breath, and see if you can stretch a little farther. Do this 5–6 times, then repeat on the other side.

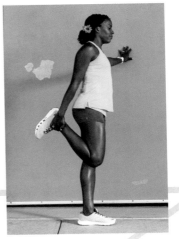

STANDING HAMSTRING STRETCH

Extend one leg just out in front of you and let the knee of the opposite leg bend as you reach forward. Try to keep your back flat.

STANDING QUAD STRETCH

Using a wall for support, stand on one leg and pull the opposite heel to your glute. Press forward through your stretched side to keep your hips and knees square.

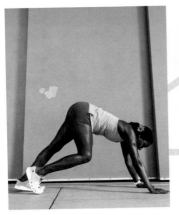

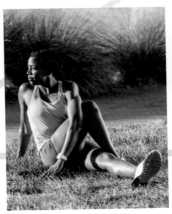

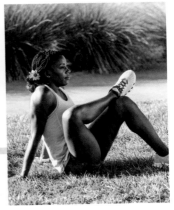

DOWNWARD DOG CALF STRETCH

Push your palms and heels into the ground, bending one knee at a time as you push the opposite heel to the ground to stretch that calf.

SEATED SPINAL ROTATION

With legs extended, cross one leg over the other and twist in the opposite direction, using your arm to push your knee in toward your chest.

SEATED GLUTE STRETCH

With knees bent, cross one leg over the other to get into a figure-4 position. Gently move closer to your stationary foot to intensify the stretch.

TOTAL-BODY STRENGTH

Because we have more time in this strength workout than we have had in other challenges, expect to push the weights heavier and the tempos to be slower!

WARM-UP

▶ Complete an easy 10-minute jog, trying to maintain a consistent pace (RPE 3 to 4) throughout.

ACTIVATION DRILLS

▶ Do 6 to 8 reps of exercises 1–5, resting 15 seconds between each exercise. Repeat for a total of 2 rounds.

1 DOUBLE HEEL SLIDE

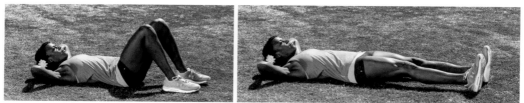

Slide both heels out and back in, keeping your core engaged and your low back flat.

2 DONKEY WHIP

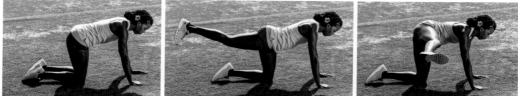

Extend one leg straight behind you; then whip it up to the side and back in a fluid, controlled motion. Engage your core and glute on the supporting side. Work both sides.

HEEL TOUCH

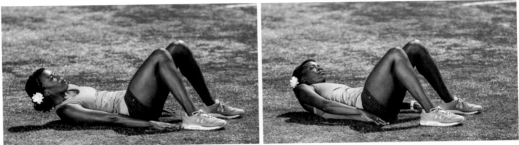

Engage your core just enough to lift your shoulders off the ground, and hold that position as you reach for your heel. Alternate side to side.

SIDE LUNGE TO KNEE DRIVE

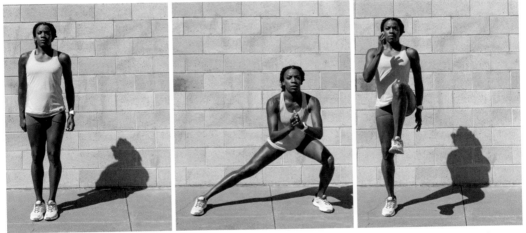

Step out to one side into a squat; then push up into a sprinter position, knee high. Work both sides.

HAMSTRING CURL

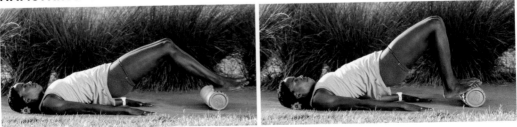

Lie on your back with the foam roller under your heels. Lift your hips up and pull your heels in until the roller reaches your toes. Continue rolling out and in.

▶ Perform each exercise in the superset to fatigue, resting for 30 seconds between exercises. Repeat for 4 rounds. Rest for 1 minute between supersets. Use 3:2:1 tempo and a weight that fatigues you in 12 to 16 reps.

1 DEADLIFT TO BENT-OVER ROW

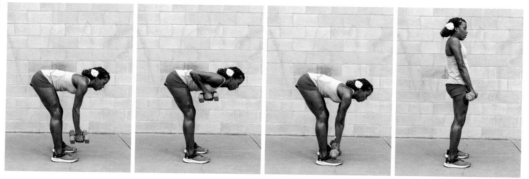

Hinge at the hips and lower the weights close to your body, until your back is parallel with the ground. Turn your palms inward. Pinch your shoulder blades together as you "row," pulling the weights up to your torso (with elbows tucked); then lower back down. Now push your ribs forward to return to standing.

CHEST PRESS

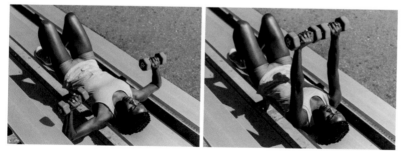

Lie on a bench, holding dumbbells straight up over your shoulders. Lower dumbbells to shoulders and press back up.

≫ CHEST PRESS, ALTERNATING

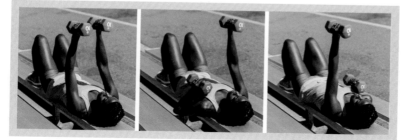

Lower one dumbbell to your shoulder and press back up as you lower the opposite dumbbell.

2 SUMO SQUAT PULSE

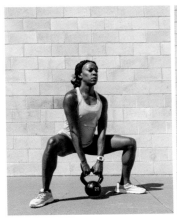 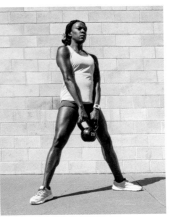

Get into a wide stance with your feet turned out and sink into a squat. Pulse up and down, and let it burn a little.

SINGLE-ARM DUMBBELL ROW

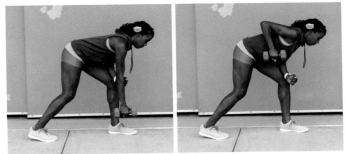

Start from a split stance, hinging forward at the hips. Hold a dumbbell in the arm opposite your forward leg and pull your elbow straight up, bringing the weight toward your torso. Keep both your back and your shoulder blades flat. Place your resting arm on the forward leg for stability. Work both sides.

3 HIP THRUST

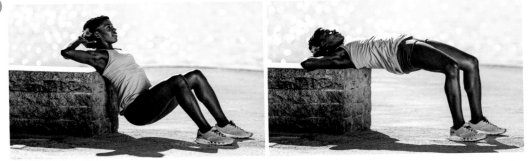

Place your shoulders on a bench and push down through your heels as you engage your glutes to raise your hips high. Pause at the top; then lower with control. Adjust your feet to be closer or farther away from your hips until you feel the work mostly in your glutes. ≫ Add weight! Hold a dumbbell with both hands across the tops of your hips.

SQUAT TO PRESS

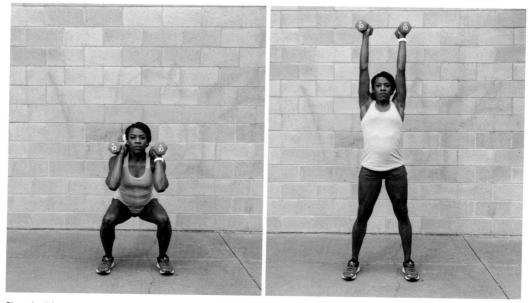

Stand with your feet shoulder-width apart, weights in front of your shoulders. Squat down and drive through your heels, pressing the weights overhead. Keep your core engaged—you shouldn't feel the load in your low back.

4 SIDE LUNGE, WITH WEIGHTS

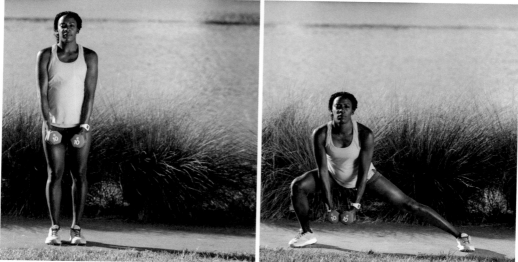

Step out to one side into a lunge; then push off back to start. Work both sides.

REAR DELT FLY

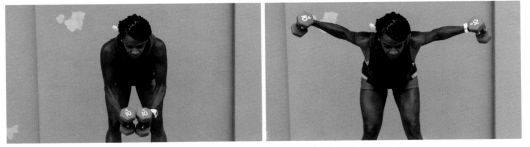

Hinge at the hips with a flat back. Squeeze your shoulder blades together to raise your arms up to shoulder height. Lower back down with control. Keep a slight bend in your elbows as you continue the movement.

FINISHER

▶ Do 30 seconds of walking lunges with weights, rest for 30 seconds, and repeat for a total of 5 to 6 rounds. Follow with the hamstring curl, performing as many reps as possible.

WALKING LUNGE

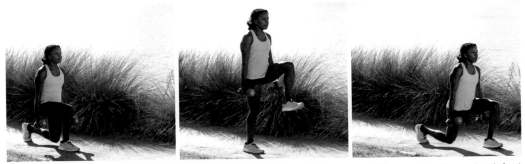

Step into a lunge, sinking down until your quad is parallel with the ground. Then push off your back foot and bring your knee high before stepping forward into a lunge on the opposite side. Let your legs do the work.

WEEKLY PROGRESSIONS

Week 2: Use a 2:1:1 tempo. Use a weight that fatigues you in 10 to 12 reps.
Week 3: Use a 3:1:1 tempo. Use a weight that fatigues you in 8 to 10 reps.
Week 4: Use a 4:1:1 tempo. Use a weight that fatigues you in 6 to 8 reps.

See p. 14 Count Your Tempo

▶ Hold each stretch for 5 seconds, take a breath, and see if you can stretch a little farther. Do this 5–6 times, then repeat on the other side.

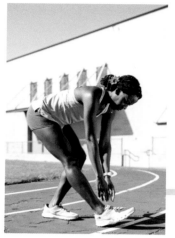

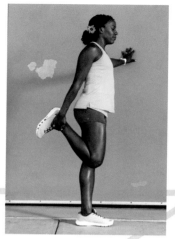

STANDING HAMSTRING STRETCH

Extend one leg just out in front of you and let the knee of the opposite leg bend as you reach forward. Try to keep your back flat.

STANDING QUAD STRETCH

Using a wall for support, stand on one leg and pull the opposite heel to your glute. Press forward through your stretched side to keep your hips and knees square.

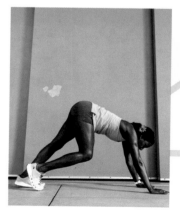

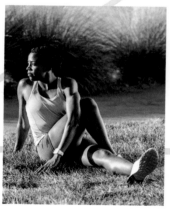

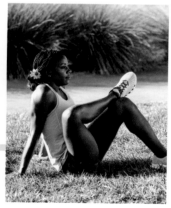

DOWNWARD DOG CALF STRETCH

Push your palms and heels into the ground, bending one knee at a time as you push the opposite heel to the ground to stretch that calf.

SEATED SPINAL ROTATION

With legs extended, cross one leg over the other and twist in the opposite direction, using your arm to push your knee in toward your chest.

SEATED GLUTE STRETCH

With knees bent, cross one leg over the other to get into a figure-4 position. Gently move closer to your stationary foot to intensify the stretch.

SPEED + POWER

Using a combination of fartleks (a Swedish term that means "speed play") and hills, this workout will improve your speed, acceleration, and ability to remain in control on both inclines and declines.

WARM-UP

▶ Complete an easy 10-minute jog, trying to maintain a consistent pace (RPE 3 to 4) throughout.

ACTIVATION DRILLS

▶ Do 6 to 8 reps of each exercise in the superset, resting 15 seconds between each round. Do 3 rounds, then the next superset.

1 REVERSE PLANK WITH LEG LIFT

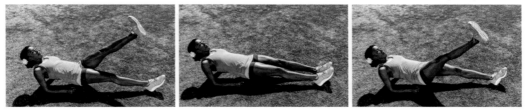

Lean back on your elbows and lift your body into plank position. Engage your core as you alternate leg lifts—only as high as you can go while holding the plank.

V-UP

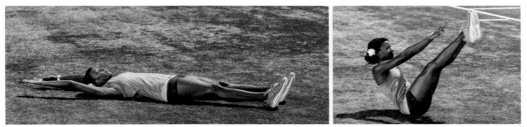

Extend your arms overhead and engage your core as you lift your legs and reach up and forward, toward your feet. Come back down with control. Keep your arms, legs, and back as straight as possible.

2 SKATER JUMP

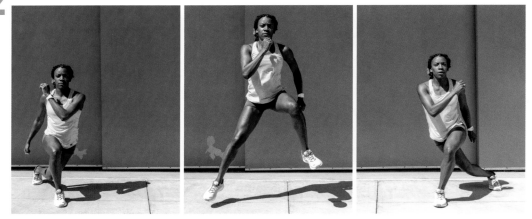

Jump from side to side. As you land, swing the inside leg behind you and touch down lightly before bounding back to the other side.

PUSH-UP SIDE KNEE HIKES

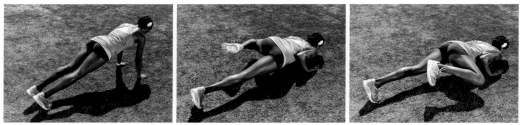

Get into a high-plank position and lower your body into a push-up. Pump your knee up to your elbow, then switch knees before pushing back up to a high plank. Keep the sequence going.

3 LATERAL BAND WALK

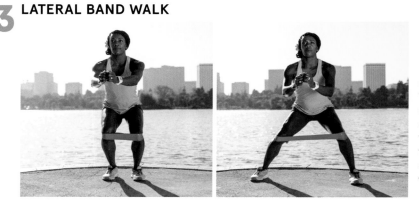

Place the band just below your knees. From a half-squat stance, step one foot out to the side and follow with the opposite foot, keeping the band taut at all times. Return in the opposite direction to work the other side.

BAND WALK

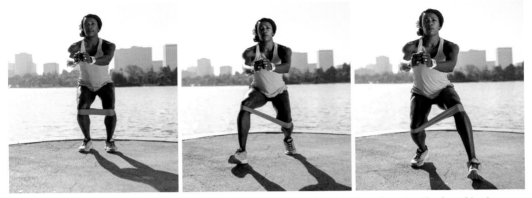

Stand with your feet shoulder-width apart and walk forward, heel-to-toe, keeping the band taut. Halfway through the reps walk backward, toe-to-heel.

RUN

FARTLEKS Run for 20 minutes, alternating between a nice, easy pace (RPE 3 to 4) and short, high-intensity sprints (RPE 9). During your run, choose an object in front of you, such as a mailbox or light post, sprint to it, and repeat.

HILLS Run up your hill of choice for 2 minutes at your 5K pace. If your hill doesn't take a full 2 minutes to climb, once you get to the top, run out the clock with the High Knees exercise, moving as fast as possible and staying on your toes. Slowly jog down the hill to recover, maintaining control rather than "breaking" with each foot strike. Repeat for a total of 3 sets.

When doing hills, focus on good form, keeping a tucked tailbone and engaging your core to help activate your power muscles for overall strength and power. Be mindful of keeping your normal running cadence (resist the urge to lengthen your strides!) and you'll take those hills faster than your little voice might be telling you that you can.

WEEKLY PROGRESSIONS
Work your way up to 5 sets on the hill runs.

See p. 62 Finding Hills Near You

▶ Hold each stretch for 5 seconds, take a breath, and see if you can stretch a little farther. Do this 5–6 times, then repeat on the other side.

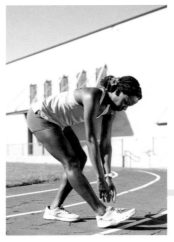

STANDING HAMSTRING STRETCH

Extend one leg just out in front of you and let the knee of the opposite leg bend as you reach forward. Try to keep your back flat.

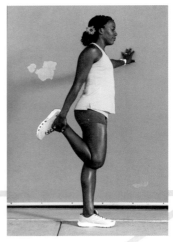

STANDING QUAD STRETCH

Using a wall for support, stand on one leg and pull the opposite heel to your glute. Press forward through your stretched side to keep your hips and knees square.

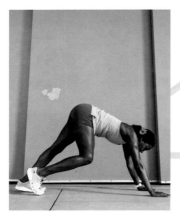

DOWNWARD DOG CALF STRETCH

Push your palms and heels into the ground, bending one knee at a time as you push the opposite heel to the ground to stretch that calf.

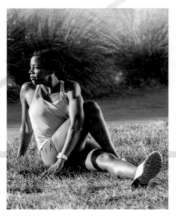

SEATED SPINAL ROTATION

With legs extended, cross one leg over the other and twist in the opposite direction, using your arm to push your knee in toward your chest.

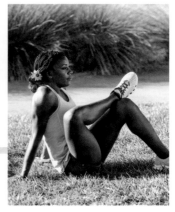

SEATED GLUTE STRETCH

With knees bent, cross one leg over the other to get into a figure-4 position. Gently move closer to your stationary foot to intensify the stretch.

HIGH-INTENSITY PLYOMETRICS

It's time to build on the plyometrics you've performed in prior challenges, increasing the amount of impact you place on your muscles' elastic components. To do so, the focus here will be on increasing jump height and the amount of single-leg work that you perform.

WARM-UP

▶ Complete an easy 10-minute jog, trying to maintain a consistent pace (RPE 3 to 4) throughout.

ACTIVATION DRILLS

▶ Do 2 sets of 6 to 8 reps of exercises 1–3 back-to-back without rest.

1 DONKEY WHIP

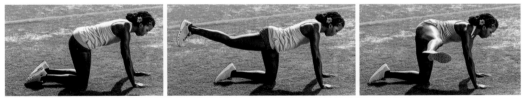

Extend one leg straight behind you; then whip it up to the side and back in a fluid, controlled motion. Engage your core and glute on the supporting side. Work both sides.

2 HEEL TOUCH

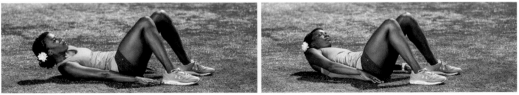

Engage your core just enough to lift your shoulders off the ground, and hold that position as you reach for your heel. Alternate side to side.

3 SIDE LUNGE TO KNEE DRIVE

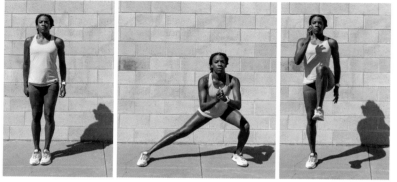

Step out to one side into a squat; then push up into a sprinter position, knee high. Work both sides.

PLYO EXERCISES

▶ Do 4 30-second sets of each exercise, resting 30 seconds between sets. Rest for 1 minute before moving on to the next exercise. Capitalize on the longer rest periods by digging deep and giving each rep everything you've got.

BOX JUMP

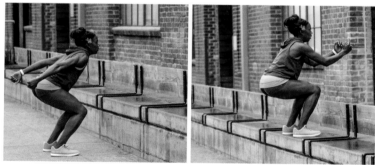

Swing your arms behind you as you squat down; then drive through your legs to explode up and forward. Land soft and step back down. Increase box height as you improve.

≫ SINGLE-LEG BOX JUMP

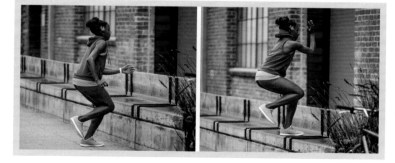

Stand on one leg and swing your arms behind you as you squat down; then drive through your leg to explode up and forward. Land soft and step back down. Work both sides.

OVERHEAD MED BALL SLAM

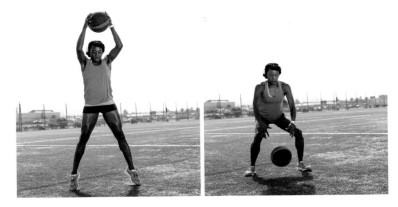

Bring the med ball overhead. Slam it straight down, catch it on the bounce, and keep on going.

LUMBERJACK MED BALL SLAM

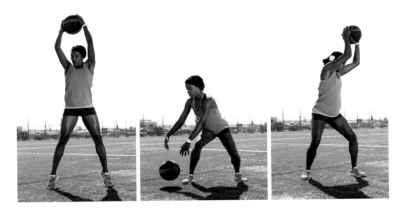

Bring the med ball overhead, slam it down to one side, catch it on the bounce, raise it overhead, and slam it down on the opposite side. Find your rhythm, moving side to side.

ROLY-POLY POWER JUMP

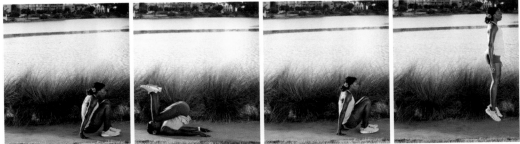

Start in a standing position, sit down, roll backward bringing your knees to chest; then quickly roll up onto your feet and power up into a jump.

SKATER JUMP

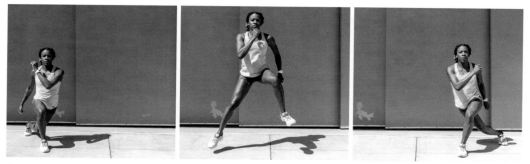

Jump from side to side. As you land, swing the inside leg behind you and touch down lightly before bounding back to the other side.

FORWARD BOUND

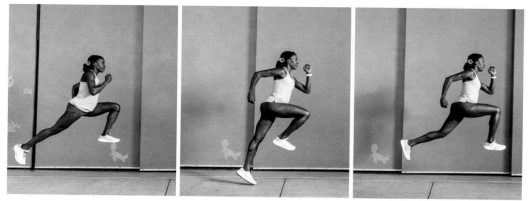

Bound forward, driving off of each foot, and landing soft.

SPLIT SQUAT JUMP

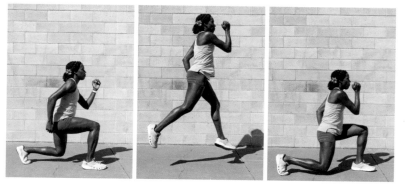

Start in a split stance and pop up. Switch your stance as you hit the height of your jump and land soft. Get your arms moving opposite your legs so you can tap that momentum.

▶ Hold each stretch for 5 seconds, take a breath, and see if you can stretch a little farther. Do this 5–6 times, then repeat on the other side.

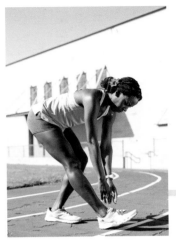

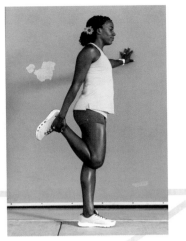

STANDING HAMSTRING STRETCH

Extend one leg just out in front of you and let the knee of the opposite leg bend as you reach forward. Try to keep your back flat.

STANDING QUAD STRETCH

Using a wall for support, stand on one leg and pull the opposite heel to your glute. Press forward through your stretched side to keep your hips and knees square.

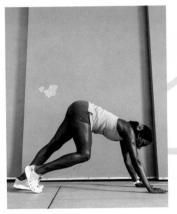

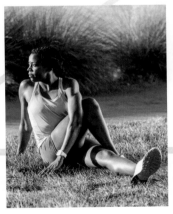

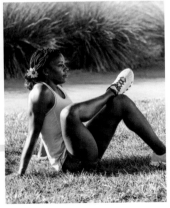

DOWNWARD DOG CALF STRETCH

Push your palms and heels into the ground, bending one knee at a time as you push the opposite heel to the ground to stretch that calf.

SEATED SPINAL ROTATION

With legs extended, cross one leg over the other and twist in the opposite direction, using your arm to push your knee in toward your chest.

SEATED GLUTE STRETCH

With knees bent, cross one leg over the other to get into a figure-4 position. Gently move closer to your stationary foot to intensify the stretch.

FLEXIBILITY + MOBILITY

This workout will feel like a cross between a strength exercise and a stretch to relieve tension; help you move in new, healthier ways; and reduce your risk of running (or everyday life) injury.

MOBILITY

▶ Perform each exercise in the superset for 30 seconds back-to-back, and repeat for three rounds. Rest for 15 seconds between supersets.

1 WALL SLIDE

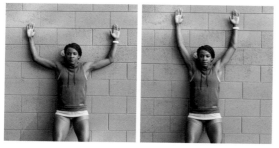

Stand with your butt, shoulders, elbows, and hands against the wall. Extend your arms up the wall, trying to limit the arch in your low back; then lower your body back down the wall.

FORWARD LEG SWING

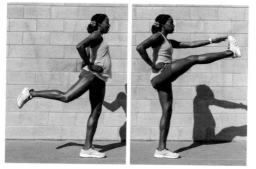

Swing one leg forward and back. Hold a wall for stability if needed. Repeat on the other side.

SIDEWAYS LEG SWING

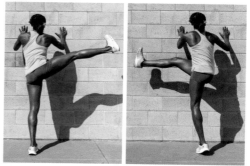

Face the wall and swing one leg from side to side. Work the other side.

2 TWISTING SUPERWOMAN

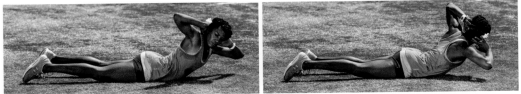

Place your hands behind your head and engage your trunk muscles to lift and twist your torso from side to side with control. Back off the lift slightly if you feel the load in your low back.

ALTERNATING SUPERWOMAN

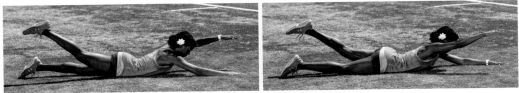

Engage your trunk muscles to lift and lower the opposing arm and leg with control; alternate sides. Back off the lift slightly if you feel the load in your low back.

STRAIGHT-LEG HIP CIRCLES

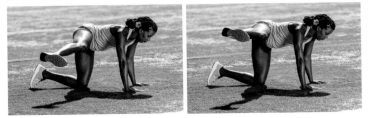

Engage your glutes to raise one leg straight out to your side. In one fluid motion, make a circle with your foot. Halfway through your reps, reverse direction. Work the other side.

3 HIP SWITCH

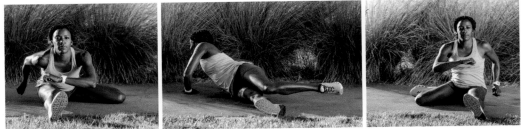

Sit with one leg extended and your other leg bent at a 90-degree angle behind you. Lean forward with the opposite arm leading the stretch. Now swing your back leg around and roll laterally into a stretch on the opposite side. Find your rhythm, moving dynamically from side to side.

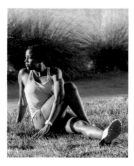

SEATED SPINAL ROTATION

With legs extended, cross one leg over the other and twist in the opposite direction, using your arm to push your knee in toward your chest. Stretch both sides.

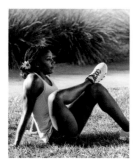

SEATED GLUTE STRETCH

With knees bent, cross one leg over the other to get into a figure-4 position. Gently move closer to your stationary foot to intensify the stretch. Stretch the other side.

COOLDOWN

▶ Stretch for 5–10 seconds and release. Repeat, maybe taking it a little farther as you exhale. After a few sets, work the other side.

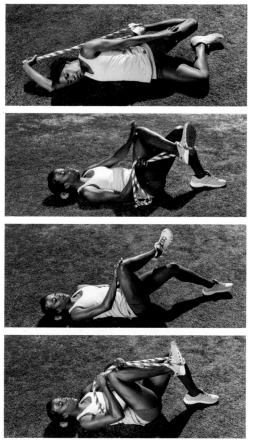

QUAD ROPE STRETCH

Lying on your side, pull your foot toward your butt, keeping it flexed. Let your knee travel behind your hips.

ABDUCTOR ROPE STRETCH

Use the rope to gently pull your foot out to one side, using your hand to keep your knee aligned with your hip.

ADDUCTOR ROPE STRETCH

Use the rope to gently pull one foot in toward your torso, using your hand to keep your knee aligned with your hip.

GLUTE ROPE STRETCH

Bring one knee in toward your chest, using the rope to deepen the stretch.

ENDURANCE

Today is all about building muscular and aerobic endurance. We aren't pushing the pace, aiming for high-intensity work, or jacking our heart rate to a high degree.

WARM-UP

▶ Complete an easy 10-minute jog, trying to maintain a consistent pace (RPE 3 to 4) throughout.

ACTIVATION DRILLS

▶ Do 6 to 8 reps of each superset, resting 15 seconds between each exercise. Repeat for a total of 2 rounds.

1 DONKEY WHIP

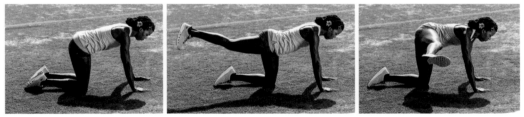

Extend one leg straight behind you; then whip it up to the side and back in a fluid, controlled motion. Engage your core and glute on the supporting side. Work both sides.

HEEL TOUCH

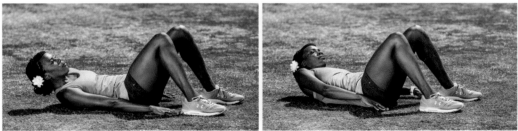

Engage your core just enough to lift your shoulders off the ground, and hold that position as you reach for your heel. Alternate side to side.

SIDE LUNGE TO KNEE DRIVE

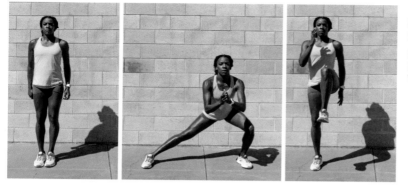

Step out to one side into a squat; then push up into a sprinter position, knee high. Work both sides.

2 LATERAL BAND WALK

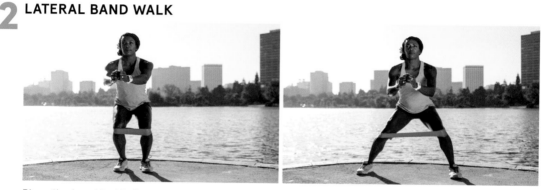

Place the band just below your knees. From a half-squat stance, step one foot out to the side and follow with the opposite foot, keeping the band taut at all times. Return in the opposite direction to work the other side.

BAND WALK

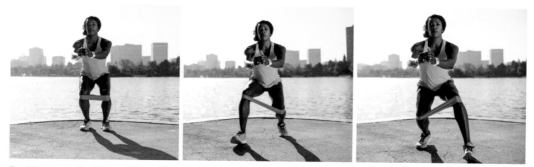

Position your feet shoulder-width apart and walk forward, heel-to-toe, keeping the band taut. Halfway through the reps walk backward, toe-to-heel.

DUCK WALK

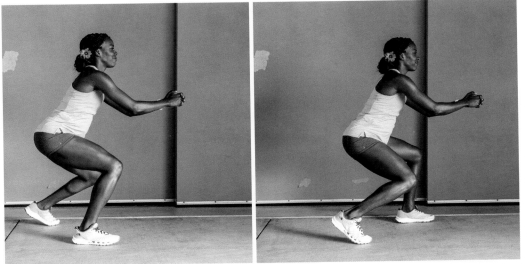

Walk forward in a squat stance, heel first, pushing through the toe. Walk backward, reversing the foot motion, rolling toe to heel.

RUN

ENDURANCE RUN Run or jog for 45 minutes. Focus on keeping a comfortable pace (RPE 4 to 5) that would allow you to carry on a conversation with a workout buddy or sing along with whatever is playing on your headphones.

WEEKLY PROGRESSIONS
Try to shave a few seconds off your pace each week. Pay attention to your breathing and form to increase your speed without increasing how hard you feel you're working. If you have a running watch or fitness tracker, try to maintain the same average heart rate from week to week. You might be surprised how much faster you can get by working smarter, not just harder!

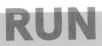

▶ Hold each stretch for 5 seconds, take a breath, and see if you can stretch a little farther. Do this 5–6 times, then repeat on the other side.

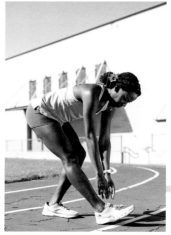

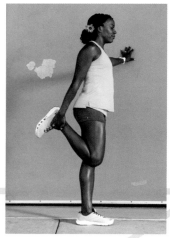

STANDING HAMSTRING STRETCH

Extend one leg just out in front of you and let the knee of the opposite leg bend as you reach forward. Try to keep your back flat.

STANDING QUAD STRETCH

Using a wall for support, stand on one leg and pull the opposite heel to your glute. Press forward through your stretched side to keep your hips and knees square.

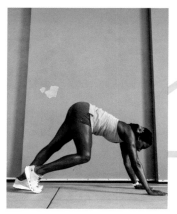

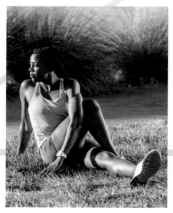

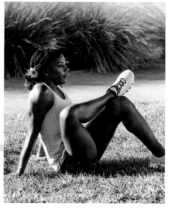

DOWNWARD DOG CALF STRETCH

Push your palms and heels into the ground, bending one knee at a time as you push the opposite heel to the ground to stretch that calf.

SEATED SPINAL ROTATION

With legs extended, cross one leg over the other and twist in the opposite direction, using your arm to push your knee in toward your chest.

SEATED GLUTE STRETCH

With knees bent, cross one leg over the other to get into a figure-4 position. Gently move closer to your stationary foot to intensify the stretch.

Challenge 9

LEVEL UP
YOUR RUNNING

One of my favorite things about running is that no matter what I've done and achieved, there is always new territory to explore and conquer. *Favorite?!?* You might be thinking that's the worst thing ever. But, as you enter this challenge, I encourage you to embrace running as a journey rather than just a finish line to cross.

Here, we will harness the mindset, running skills, strength, and endurance that you've already built throughout past challenges to take you in new directions. You'll play with threshold intervals, and learn how to take downhills in stride, and your long runs will be longer than ever. It's going to be challenging, which is why I've taken the liberty of scheduling your recovery for the days that you'll need it most. Use your improved running fitness to run a faster 5K or test your legs on a 10K. Find a race that's six weeks out or simply repeat your Benchmark Run at the end of the challenge.

But it should also be fun! Enjoy your workouts, explore new running paths, celebrate your running prowess, and take a sweaty selfie. Welcome to your next level!

Bonus!

Do a Benchmark Run (p. 221) before starting this challenge so you can see how far you have come.

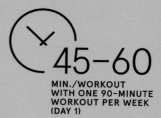

45–60

MIN./WORKOUT
WITH ONE 90-MINUTE
WORKOUT PER WEEK
(DAY 1)

5 days per week for *6 weeks*

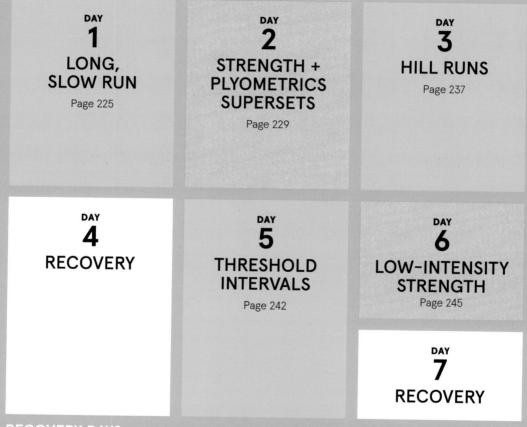

DAY 1
LONG, SLOW RUN
Page 225

DAY 2
STRENGTH + PLYOMETRICS SUPERSETS
Page 229

DAY 3
HILL RUNS
Page 237

DAY 4
RECOVERY

DAY 5
THRESHOLD INTERVALS
Page 242

DAY 6
LOW-INTENSITY STRENGTH
Page 245

DAY 7
RECOVERY

RECOVERY DAYS   In past challenges, you've chosen your own recovery days. The first few days of this challenge are so challenging that it's worth taking a day off as scheduled, at least in Week 1. If you do want to get a little recovery work in in subsequent weeks, check out the **Foam Rolling** and **Mobility** routines in the Appendix (p. 270).

EQUIPMENT   Running shoes ▪ dumbbells ▪ 2 resistance bands (1 short, 1 long) ▪ medicine ball ▪ foam roller

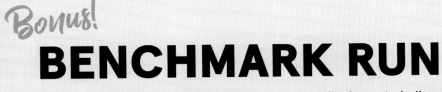

Bonus!

BENCHMARK RUN

By now, you're moving faster than ever, so just like in past challenges, we are going to keep track of your current pace. This workout will take you through a gentle warm-up, activation drills, and a 5K time trial. If you don't have a race on your calendar, at the end of this challenge, do it again to see just how much you've gained!

WARM-UP

▶ Complete an easy 10-minute jog to get your heart rate up and muscles ready to go. Aim for an RPE of 3 to 4. Then perform 10 reps of the Forward Bound.

FORWARD BOUND

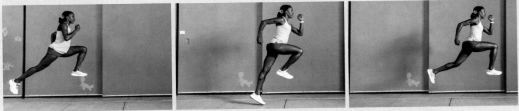

Bound forward, driving off of each foot, and landing soft.

ACTIVATION DRILLS

▶ Do 6 to 8 reps of each exercise, resting 15 seconds between them.

SPLIT-LEG CRUNCH

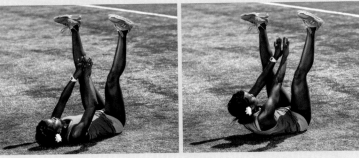

With legs extended, engage your abs to raise your shoulders and reach; then come back down with control. Keep your back flat and legs still.

SPLIT-LEG CROSS-TOE TOUCH

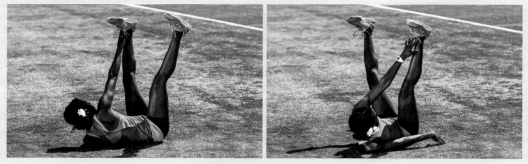

Engage your abs to raise your shoulders and reach your hand to the opposite foot; then come back down with control. Alternate sides, keeping your back flat and legs still.

ALTERNATING SUPERWOMAN

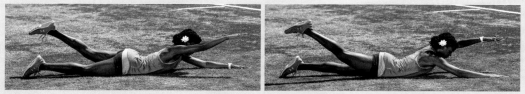

Engage your trunk muscles to lift and lower the opposing arm and leg with control; alternate sides. Back off the lift slightly if you feel the load in your low back.

Consistency

FLOWER POWER

We all know that it takes a few days to create a bad habit and far longer to break it, let alone replace it with a good habit. When you commit to a routine, you create a habit of consistency that sets you up for success. Make room for more healthy patterns in your routine: Leave a note on the mirror to remind you to drink a glass of water first thing in the morning. Plan to work out on the first day of every month or the first day of every week. Reset your day, week, or month with a positive behavior pattern, even when life has gotten the best of you.

Counter the tendency to be obsessive or rigid with a good measure of flexibility—because even a good thing can be taken too far. These patterns of consistency make the task of taking care of yourself second nature: Before you run, you warm up with a few key exercises; before you lift weights, you activate the muscles.

Balance your health and fitness with other things that have a regular place in your routine, like passion projects, hobbies, family, and friends. A regular dose of these good things will keep you from resenting your pursuits when things flip upside down.

A-SKIP

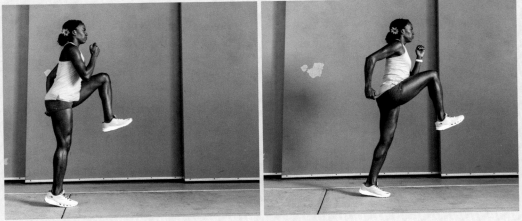

Hop-skip with high knees, swinging your arms to keep momentum.

B-SKIP

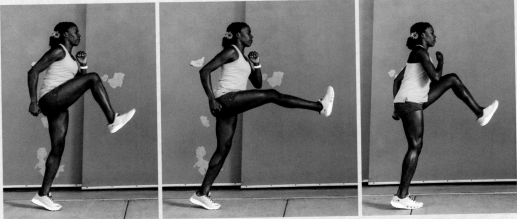

Hop-skip, engaging your glute to pull your knee up (like the A-Skip), then swing your leg forward to extension. Move your arms for momentum.

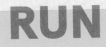

TIME TRIAL Give it all you've got! Run 3.1 miles (RPE 7 to 8). Using a running watch or following a set 5K course, time how fast you can run 3.1 miles.

▶ Hold each stretch for 5 seconds, take a breath, and see if you can stretch a little farther. Do this 5–6 times, then repeat on the other side.

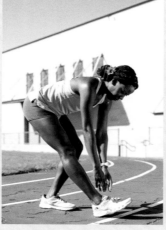

STANDING HAMSTRING STRETCH

Extend one leg just out in front of you and let the knee of the opposite leg bend as you reach forward. Try to keep your back flat.

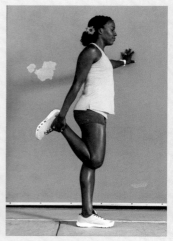

STANDING QUAD STRETCH

Using a wall for support, stand on one leg and pull the opposite heel to your glute. Press forward through your stretched side to keep your hips and knees square.

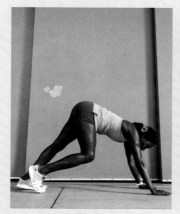

DOWNWARD DOG CALF STRETCH

Push your palms and heels into the ground, bending one knee at a time as you push the opposite heel to the ground to stretch that calf.

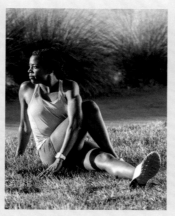

SEATED SPINAL ROTATION

With legs extended, cross one leg over the other and twist in the opposite direction, using your arm to push your knee in toward your chest.

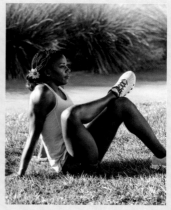

SEATED GLUTE STRETCH

With knees bent, cross one leg over the other to get into a figure-4 position. Gently move closer to your stationary foot to intensify the stretch.

LONG, SLOW RUN

Today is all about building muscular and aerobic endurance—spending a record amount of time on your feet. We aren't pushing the pace, aiming for high-intensity work, or jacking our heart rate to a high degree. Keep things relaxed—listen to some music or your favorite podcast or just zone out.

WARM-UP

▶ Complete an extremely easy 10-minute jog, trying to maintain a consistent pace (RPE 3 to 4) throughout.

ACTIVATION DRILLS

▶ Do 6 to 8 reps of exercises 1–5, resting 15 seconds between each exercise. Repeat for a total of 2 rounds.

1 DONKEY WHIP

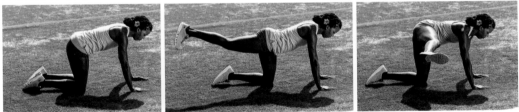

Extend one leg straight behind you; then whip it up to the side and back in a fluid, controlled motion. Engage your core and glute on the supporting side. Work both sides.

2 DOUBLE HEEL SLIDE

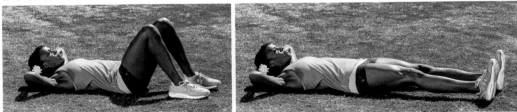

Slide both heels out and back in, keeping your core engaged and your low back flat.

3 SIDE LUNGE TO KNEE DRIVE

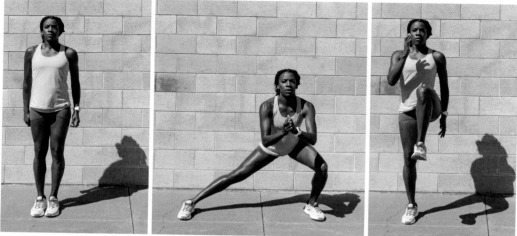

Step out to one side into a squat; then push up into a sprinter position, knee high. Work both sides.

4 LATERAL BAND WALK

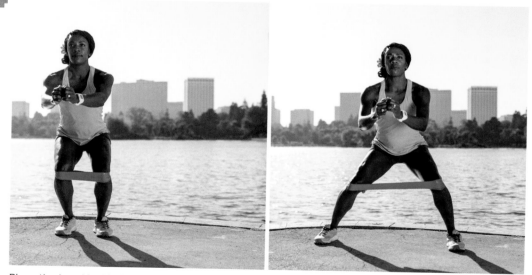

Place the band just below your knees. From a half-squat stance, step one foot out to the side and follow with the opposite foot, keeping the band taut at all times. Return in the opposite direction to work the opposite side.

5 BAND WALK

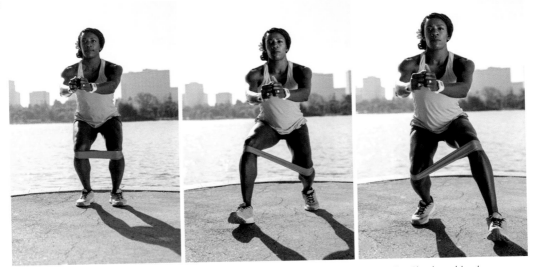

Position your feet shoulder-width apart and walk forward, heel-to-toe, keeping the band taut. Halfway through the reps walk backward, toe-to-heel.

RUN

LONG, SLOW RUN Run or jog for up to 75 minutes, starting with the longest distance you've recently and consistently ran. Focus on keeping a comfortable pace (RPE 4 to 5) that would allow you to carry on a conversation with a workout buddy or sing along with whatever is playing on your headphones.

WEEKLY PROGRESSIONS: + 0.5 MILE / 5 MINUTES

As you feel comfortable, add a half mile or 5 minutes onto your long-run distance each week or every two weeks. Work toward 90 minutes. Don't increase your weekly mileage by more than 10 percent in a given week or you run the risk of overtraining, RED-S, and injury.

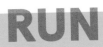

▶ Hold each stretch for 5 seconds, take a breath, and see if you can stretch a little farther. Do this 5–6 times, then repeat on the other side.

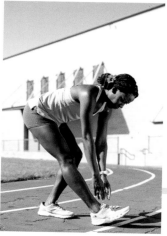

STANDING HAMSTRING STRETCH

Extend one leg just out in front of you and let the knee of the opposite leg bend as you reach forward. Try to keep your back flat.

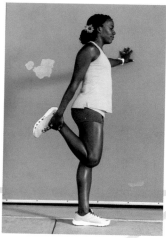

STANDING QUAD STRETCH

Using a wall for support, stand on one leg and pull the opposite heel to your glute. Press forward through your stretched side to keep your hips and knees square.

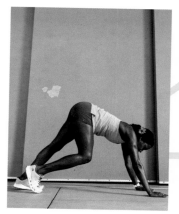

DOWNWARD DOG CALF STRETCH

Push your palms and heels into the ground, bending one knee at a time as you push the opposite heel to the ground to stretch that calf.

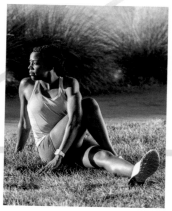

SEATED SPINAL ROTATION

With legs extended, cross one leg over the other and twist in the opposite direction, using your arm to push your knee in toward your chest.

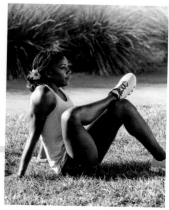

SEATED GLUTE STRETCH

With knees bent, cross one leg over the other to get into a figure-4 position. Gently move closer to your stationary foot to intensify the stretch.

STRENGTH + PLYOMETRICS SUPERSETS

Combine traditional resistance exercises with high-loaded, run-mimicking plyometrics to build phenomenal strength and power.

WARM-UP

▶ Complete an easy 10-minute jog, trying to maintain a consistent pace (RPE 3 to 4) throughout.

ACTIVATION DRILLS

▶ Do 6 to 8 reps of exercises 1–4, resting 15 seconds between each exercise. Repeat for a total of 2 rounds.

1 DONKEY WHIP

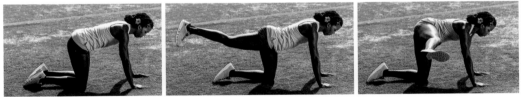

Extend one leg straight behind you; then whip it up to the side and back in a fluid, controlled motion. Engage your core and glute on the supporting side. Work both sides.

2 HEEL TOUCH

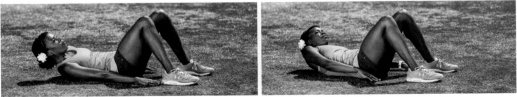

Engage your core just enough to lift your shoulders off the ground, and hold that position as you reach for your heel. Alternate side to side.

3 SIDE LUNGE TO KNEE DRIVE

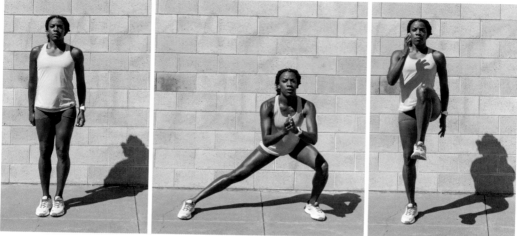

Step out to one side into a squat; then push up into a sprinter position, knee high. Work both sides.

4 SINGLE-LEG POWER-UP

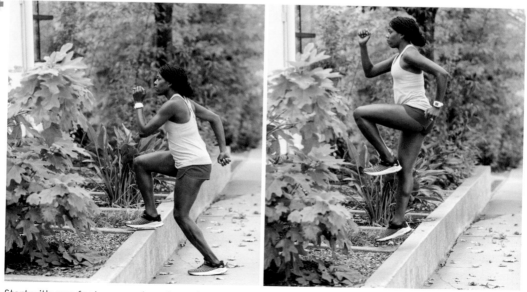

Start with one foot up on a bench or step. Drive through that leg as you explode up and raise your opposite knee toward your chest; then land soft and step back down. Keep a steady rhythm, moving your arms opposite your legs to create momentum. Work both sides.

▶ Do each exercise in the superset for 30 seconds, then rest for 30 seconds.
Complete 6 sets, resting for 1 minute between supersets.

1 SINGLE-LEG BOX JUMP

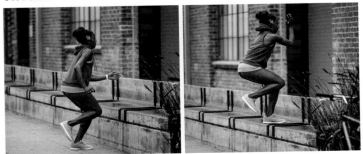

Stand on one leg and swing your arms behind you as you squat down; then drive through your leg to explode up and forward. Land soft and step back down. Increase box height as you improve. Work both sides.

« BOX JUMP

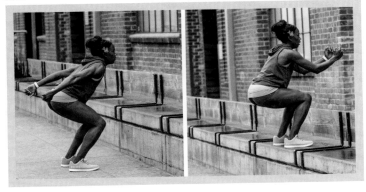

Swing your arms behind you as you squat down; then drive through your legs to explode up and forward. Land soft and step back down.

SINGLE-ARM DUMBBELL ROW

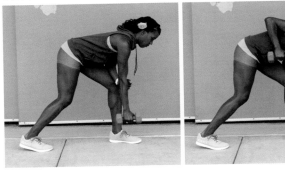

Start from a split stance, hinging forward at the hips. Hold a dumbbell in the arm opposite your forward leg and pull your elbow straight up, bringing the weight toward your torso. Keep both your back and your shoulder blades flat. Place your resting arm on the forward leg for stability. Work both sides.

2 ROLY-POLY POWER JUMP

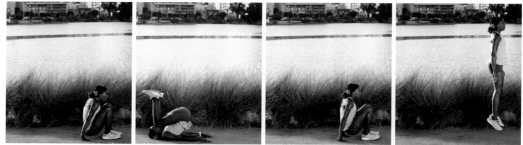

Start in a standing position, sit down, roll backward bringing your knees to chest; then quickly roll up onto your feet and power up into a jump.

PUSH-UP

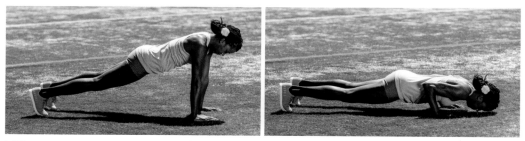

With your hands under your shoulders, squeeze your back, abs, and glutes to hold your body in a straight line. Lower your body to the ground, keeping your elbows tucked; then press back up.

3 SKATER JUMP

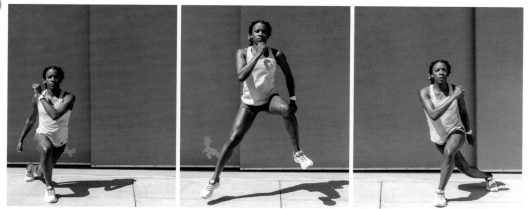

Jump from side to side. As you land, swing the inside leg behind you and touch down lightly before bounding back to the other side.

REAR DELT FLY

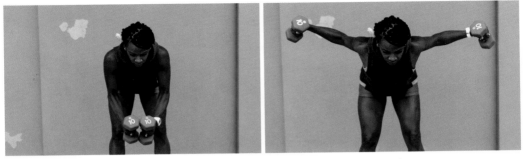

Hinge at the hips with a flat back. Squeeze your shoulder blades together to raise your arms up to shoulder height. Lower back down with control. Keep a slight bend in your elbows as you continue the movement.

 ## SPLIT SQUAT JUMP

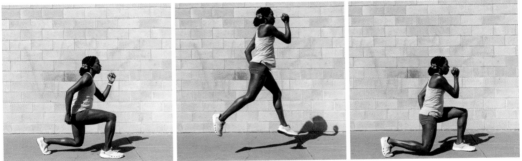

Start in a split stance and pop up. Switch your stance as you hit the height of your jump and land soft. Get your arms moving opposite your legs so you can tap that momentum.

OVERHEAD TRICEPS EXTENSION

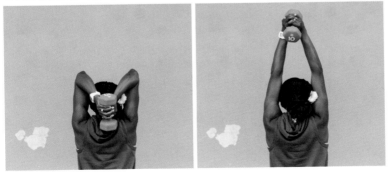

Hold the weight overhead, arms extended, and lower it with control. Keep your elbows tucked and your core strong to avoid loading your low back.

5 FORWARD BOUND

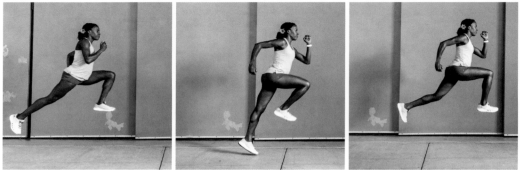

Bound forward, driving off of each foot, and landing soft.

SUMO SQUAT WITH PRESS

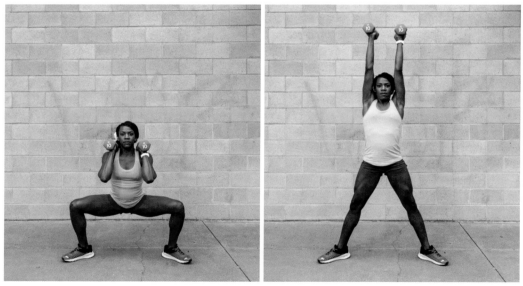

Get into a wide sumo stance, toes pointed outward and weights in front of your shoulders. Squat down and drive through your heels, pressing the weights overhead. Keep your core engaged—you shouldn't feel the load in your low back.

▶ Do as many reps as possible of each exercise in this med ball superset in 1 minute. Alternate between the two moves however you like! Rest for 30 seconds; then repeat for a total of 3 rounds.

6 OVERHEAD MED BALL SLAM

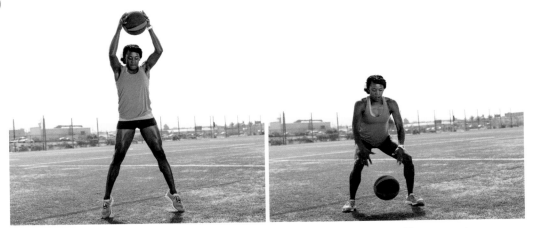

Bring the med ball overhead. Slam it straight down, catch it on the bounce, and keep on going.

LUMBERJACK MED BALL SLAM

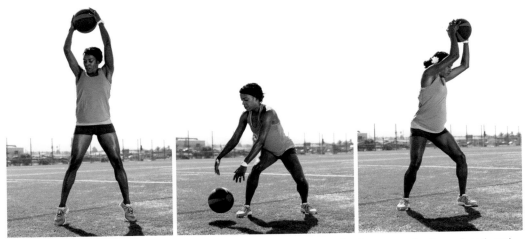

Bring the med ball overhead, slam it down to one side, catch it on the bounce, raise it overhead, and slam it down on the opposite side. Find your rhythm, moving side to side.

▶ Hold each stretch for 5 seconds, take a breath, and see if you can stretch a little farther. Do this 5–6 times, then repeat on the other side.

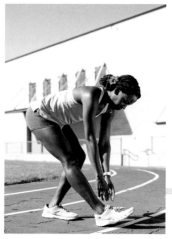

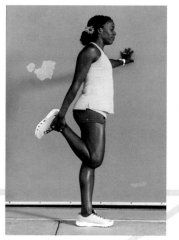

STANDING HAMSTRING STRETCH

Extend one leg just out in front of you and let the knee of the opposite leg bend as you reach forward. Try to keep your back flat.

STANDING QUAD STRETCH

Using a wall for support, stand on one leg and pull the opposite heel to your glute. Press forward through your stretched side to keep your hips and knees square.

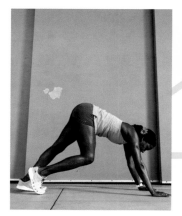

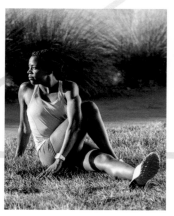

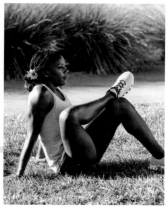

DOWNWARD DOG CALF STRETCH

Push your palms and heels into the ground, bending one knee at a time as you push the opposite heel to the ground to stretch that calf.

SEATED SPINAL ROTATION

With legs extended, cross one leg over the other and twist in the opposite direction, using your arm to push your knee in toward your chest.

SEATED GLUTE STRETCH

With knees bent, cross one leg over the other to get into a figure-4 position. Gently move closer to your stationary foot to intensify the stretch.

HILL RUNS

Improve your speed, acceleration, and muscle recruitment with inclines. On the declines, you'll work your quads, increasing their capacity to take on load.

WARM-UP

▶ Complete an easy 10-minute jog, trying to maintain a consistent pace (RPE 3 to 4) throughout.

ACTIVATION DRILLS

▶ Do 6 to 8 reps of each exercise in the superset. Rest 15 seconds, then repeat the superset for a total of 3 rounds.

1 LATERAL BAND WALK

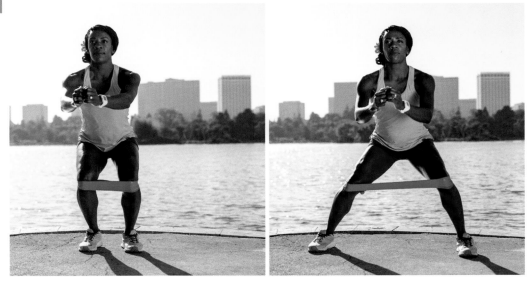

Place the band just below your knees. From a half-squat stance, step one foot out to the side and follow with the opposite foot, keeping the band taut at all times. Return in the opposite direction to work the other side.

BAND WALK

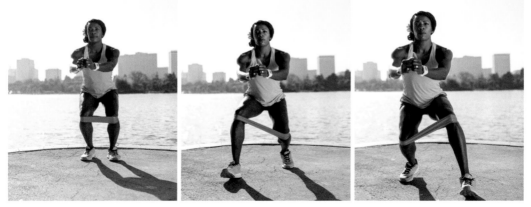

Position your feet shoulder-width apart and walk forward, heel-to-toe, keeping the band taut. Halfway through the reps walk backward, toe-to-heel.

2 SKATER JUMP

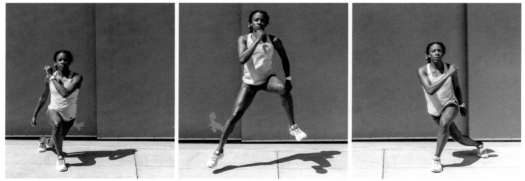

Jump from side to side. As you land, swing the inside leg behind you and touch down lightly before bounding back to the other side.

SINGLE-LEG DEADLIFT TO KNEE DRIVE

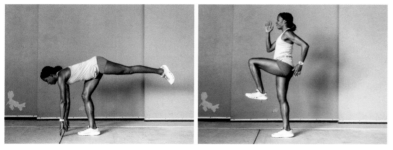

Balance on one leg, extending the opposite leg straight behind you, and tip forward. Keep your back flat and pendulum-swing your leg back up to a high-knee stance. Work both sides.

3 HURDLE WALK-OVERS

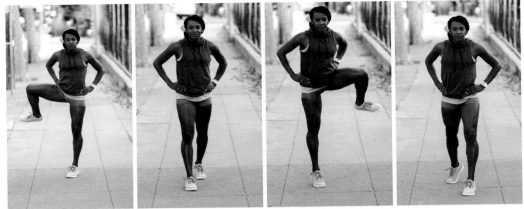

Lift one leg up and out to the side as if you were stepping over a hurdle and moving forward; continue alternating legs.

SIDE HURDLE

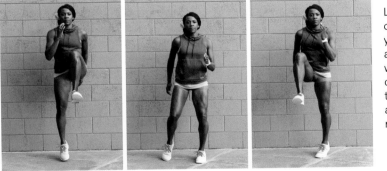

Lift one leg up and step out to the side as if you are stepping over a hurdle, and follow with the trailing leg coming up and over the hurdle. Keep it going, and halfway through the reps, switch direction.

4 A-SKIP

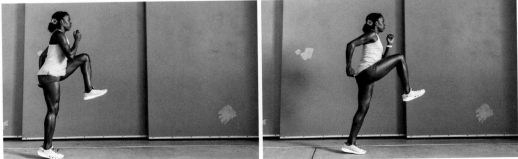

Hop-skip with high knees, swinging your arms to keep momentum.

B-SKIP

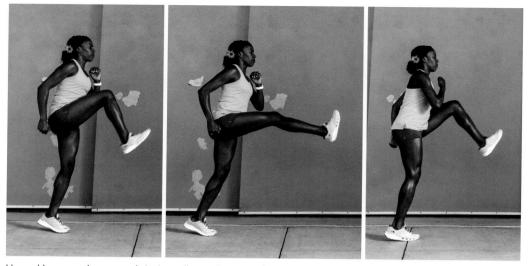

Hop-skip, engaging your glute to pull your knee up (like the A-Skip), then swing your leg forward to extension. Move your arms for momentum.

RUN

HILLS Sprint up a hill for 30, 45, and then 60 seconds (RPE 7 to 8). Between each sprint, run at moderate intensity down the hill, keeping your body perpendicular to the ground, embracing the free speed, and maintaining control rather than "breaking" with each foot strike; then rest for 1 minute. Repeat for a total of 3 sets, resting for 3 minutes between each.

When doing hills, focus on good form, keeping a tucked tailbone and engaging your core to help you activate your power muscles for overall strength and power.

WEEKLY PROGRESSIONS

Gradually increase the number of sets according to your current training goals or level up your hill intervals to 45, 60, and then 75 seconds.

5K Goal: 4–5 sets
10K Goal: 6–7 sets
Half-Marathon Goal: 8–10 sets

See p. 62 Finding Hills Near You

▶ Hold each stretch for 5 seconds, take a breath, and see if you can stretch a little farther. Do this 5–6 times, then repeat on the other side.

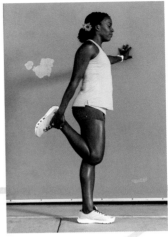

STANDING HAMSTRING STRETCH

Extend one leg just out in front of you and let the knee of the opposite leg bend as you reach forward. Try to keep your back flat.

STANDING QUAD STRETCH

Using a wall for support, stand on one leg and pull the opposite heel to your glute. Press forward through your stretched side to keep your hips and knees square.

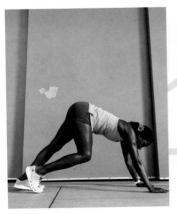

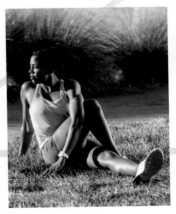

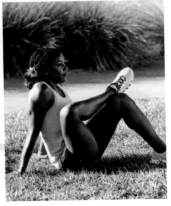

DOWNWARD DOG CALF STRETCH

Push your palms and heels into the ground, bending one knee at a time as you push the opposite heel to the ground to stretch that calf.

SEATED SPINAL ROTATION

With legs extended, cross one leg over the other and twist in the opposite direction, using your arm to push your knee in toward your chest.

SEATED GLUTE STRETCH

With knees bent, cross one leg over the other to get into a figure-4 position. Gently move closer to your stationary foot to intensify the stretch.

THRESHOLD INTERVALS

This is where it gets real. Threshold intervals are performed at an intensity where aerobic metabolism can't churn out all of the energy you need, so anaerobic metabolism kicks in, your breathing changes, and you can no longer carry on a conversation. That's the cool thing about thresholds: You can literally feel them happen.

ACTIVATION DRILLS

▶ Spend 1 minute on each foam rolling movement.

GLUTE ROLL

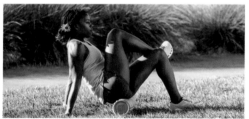

Cross one leg into a figure-4 position and roll out the glute of the stationary leg. Switch sides.

CALF ROLL

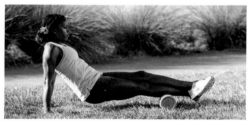

Roll out your calf muscle, using your opposite leg to go a little deeper. Roll out both sides.

UPPER-BACK ROLL

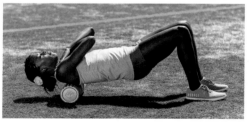

Position a foam roller under your shoulders and lift your hips. Move your feet to shift the roller up and down your back.

HIP FLEXOR ROLL

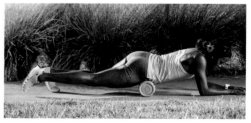

Stabilize yourself with one foot and gently roll out your hip flexor on the opposite leg. Roll out the other side.

▶ Do 6 to 8 reps of each exercise, resting 15 seconds between them.

DONKEY KICK TO FIRE HYDRANT

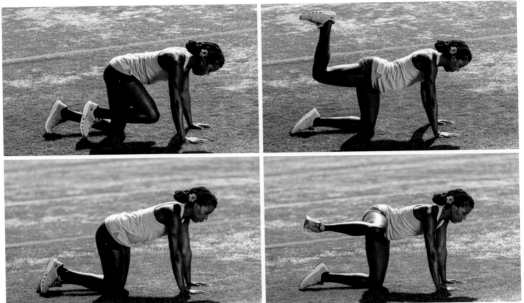

Get on all fours, and use your glutes to raise your foot up behind you and lower it back down with control. Then lift the same leg out laterally and lower with control. Engage your core to keep your back flat and feel the glutes burn, even on the stationary leg. Work both sides.

STRAIGHT-LEG HIP CIRCLES

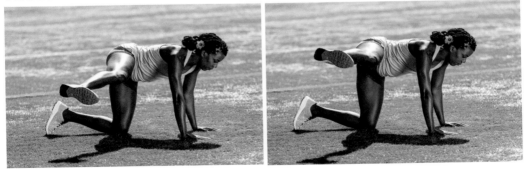

Engage your glutes to raise one leg straight out to your side. In one fluid motion, make a circle with your foot. Halfway through your reps, reverse direction. Work the other side.

WALK THE PLANK

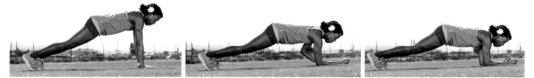

Move from a high plank to a low plank and back up again, keeping the movement going. Then switch it up to lead the up-down movement with the opposite arm. ◄ To make this easier, drop to your knees.

SUPERWOMAN

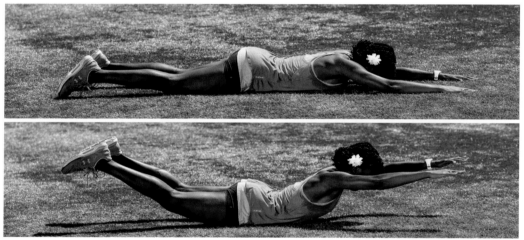

Extend your arms and engage your trunk muscles to lift your arms and legs; then lower back down with control. Back off the lift slightly if you feel the load in your low back.

RUN

INTERVALS Perform the following intervals at your threshold pace (RPE 7).

Weeks 1 + 2:
1 mile (1,600 meters)
¾ mile (1,200 meters)
½ mile (800 meters)
¼ mile (400 meters)

Walk for 3 minutes between each threshold interval.

Weeks 3 + 4: 4 × ¼ mile (400 meters

Walk for 2 minutes between each threshold interval.

Weeks 5 + 6: 12 × ⅛ mile (200 meters)

Walk for 1 minute between each threshold interval.

LOW-INTENSITY STRENGTH

This low-intensity strength workout will get the blood flowing and your muscles working through their full range of motion to improve recovery without adding to fatigue.

▶ **Spend 1 minute with each foam rolling movement.**

GLUTE ROLL

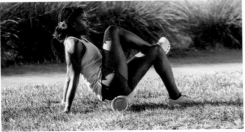

Cross one leg into a figure-4 position and roll out the glute of the stationary leg. Switch sides.

CALF ROLL

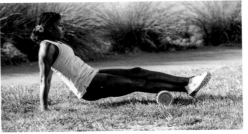

Roll out your calf muscle, using your opposite leg to go a little deeper. Switch sides.

UPPER-BACK ROLL

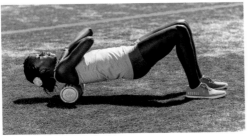

Position a foam roller under your shoulders and lift your hips. Move your feet to shift the roller up and down your back.

HIP FLEXOR ROLL

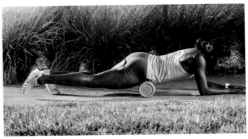

Stabilize yourself with one foot and gently roll out your hip flexor on the opposite leg. Switch sides.

▶ Do 8 to 12 reps of the exercises in each superset back-to-back. Rest for 30 seconds; then repeat for a total of 4 rounds. Rest for 30 seconds between supersets.

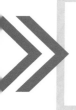

WEEKLY PROGRESSIONS
Week 2: Use a 2:1:1 tempo.
Week 3: Use a 2:2:1 tempo.
Week 4: Use a 3:1:1 tempo.
Week 5, 6: Use a 3:2:1 tempo.

1 LATERAL BAND WALK

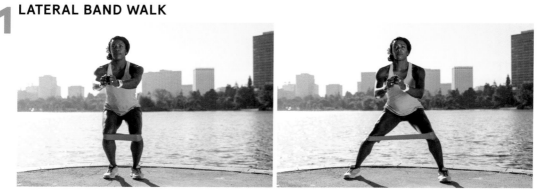

Place the band just below your knees. From a half-squat stance, step one foot out to the side and follow with the opposite foot, keeping the band taut at all times. Return in the opposite direction to work the other side.

BAND WALK

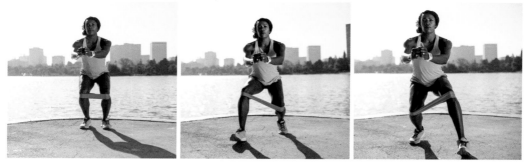

Position your feet shoulder-width apart and walk forward, heel-to-toe, keeping the band taut. Halfway through the reps walk backward, toe-to-heel.

2 HIP LIFT

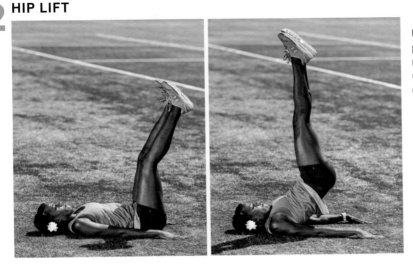

Use your core to push your hips and reach your feet upward. Come back down with control.

REVERSE PLANK WITH LATERAL EXTENSION

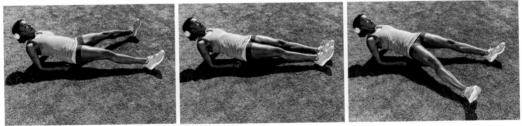

Lean back on your elbows and lift your body into plank position. Engage your core as you lift one leg out and in. Alternate sides.

3 STRAIGHT-LEG HIP CIRCLES

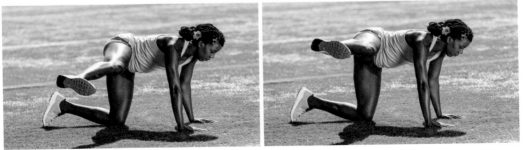

Engage your glutes to raise one leg straight out to your side. In one fluid motion, make a circle with your foot. Halfway through your reps, reverse direction. Work the other side.

LOW-INTENSITY STRENGTH

I, Y, AND T RAISES

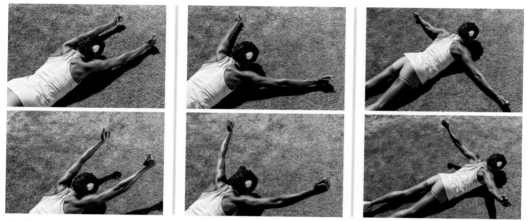

Lie down and squeeze your shoulder blades together to raise and lower your arms overhead in an "I" position, slow and controlled. Move from your shoulders, with your thumbs leading the way. Repeat to get in your Y and T raises.

4 BEAR CRAWL

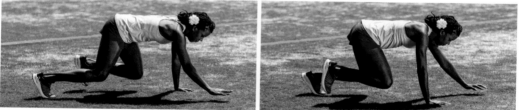

Come to your hands and the balls of your feet, and step forward with one hand and the opposite foot; then step with the opposing hand and foot. Keep your core engaged, back flat, and butt down. Halfway through the reps, move backward.

LATERAL BEAR CRAWL

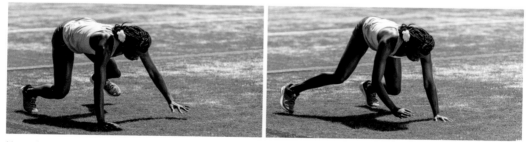

Now step to the side with one hand and the adjacent foot; then follow with the opposing hand and foot. Keep your core engaged, back flat, and butt down. Halfway through the reps, move back in the opposite direction.

Challenge 10

12 HOLY DAYS &
8 CRAZY NIGHTS

Every year, it feels like my calendar skips straight from Thanksgiving to New Year's Day! Whatever your traditions, shopping list, party schedule, baking recipes, and end-of-year deadlines, I'm guessing that your holidays are pretty hectic. So, heading into the holidays, of course you're going to feel a little *more* crazy and a bit unsure of how you're going to make it all happen.

In past years, maybe you've sacrificed some or all of your exercise routine because you felt like something had to give. Maybe you've said, "I'll start again in January." Well, next year, you won't have to start again. You'll just keep going.

That's because this challenge is all about gentle consistency and giving your mind, body, and spirit the attention they deserve, no matter the season. If you're coming off of Challenges 8 and 9, this is your opportunity to focus on maintaining your fitness with some dedicated recovery work. If you're relatively new to running, but this challenge's holiday theme caught your attention, rest assured that this workout program fits all fitness levels.

During the challenge's 12 holy days and 8 crazy nights, we'll cycle through four workouts. Feel free to schedule in some active recovery as needed, but shoot for a 12-day and 8-day streak over the course of the month.

So exhale the holiday crazies, breathe in the twinkly lights, and know that this challenge is all about giving yourself the gift of exactly what you need.

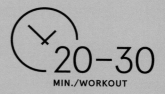

20–30
MIN./WORKOUT

4 workouts to build both a
12-day and an 8-day fitness streak

DAY **1** **LADDER RUN** Page 251	**DAY** **2** **TOTAL-BODY** **STRENGTH + MOBILITY** Page 255
DAY **3** **CORE CIRCUIT** Page 261	**DAY** **4** **ACTIVATION** Page 263

If you are short on time, drop 1–2 circuits.

RECOVERY DAYS You can add recovery days throughout and/or in between the mini-challenges. If you do want to get a little recovery work in, check out the **Foam Rolling** and **Mobility** routines in the Appendix (p. 270).

EQUIPMENT Running shoes ▪ dumbbells ▪ 2 resistance bands (1 short, 1 long) ▪ foam roller

LADDER RUN

Ladders are a fun way to reap the mind- and body-benefits of running at lots of intensities. In this one, your speed will climb—and then come back down—while the amount of time you spend at each intensity will lower, then pop back up. Don't worry about your actual pace, though. The goal is to really tune in to yourself and base every movement on what you *feel*.

WARM-UP

▶ Complete an easy 5-minute walk-jog, trying to maintain a consistent pace (RPE 3 to 4) throughout.

ACTIVATION DRILLS

▶ Do 6 reps of exercises 1–5 back-to-back without rest. Repeat for a total of 3 rounds, resting for 15 seconds between each round.

1 ALTERNATING HEEL SLIDE

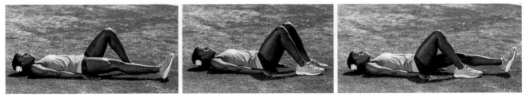

Lie down with your core engaged and your lower back flat on the ground. Slide your heel out and back in. Alternate sides.

≫ DOUBLE HEEL SLIDE

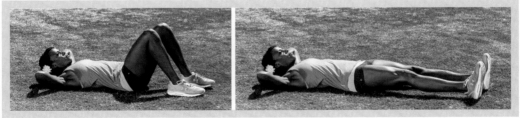

Slide both heels out and back in, keeping your core engaged and your low back flat.

2 CRUNCH TWIST

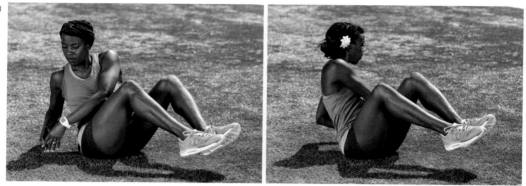

Engage your core and lift your feet off the ground, balancing on your butt. Rotate your torso as you twist from side to side, tracking your hands with your eyes. ⟫ Hold a med ball.

3 REVERSE PLANK ▶ Hold 20–30 seconds for each set.

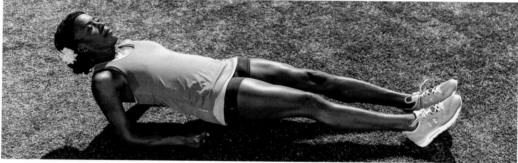

Lean back onto your elbows and engage your glutes, core, and back to hold your body in a straight line.

Redirection

FLOWER POWER

The path to success is hardly straight. Why do you think cars have steering wheels? Plan on twists and turns, even roadblocks and dead ends. Don't consider these a sign that it's time to quit—instead be open to taking an alternate route. Consider it an opportunity to hone your flexibility and practice perseverance.

In your pursuit of a fitness streak, you will have workouts that downright suck—that is to say, workouts where you came up short, sluggish, or gasping for a breath. Take some time to regroup, and write down what might have contributed to the suck—whether in the lead-up, during the workout, or afterward. Identify which of these contributing factors you can control, and steer your way around them as you power on.

4 HIP CIRCLES

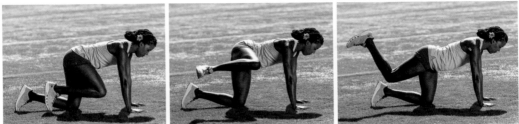

From an all-fours position, keep your core engaged as you lift your knee first out to the side, then around and behind you, and then forward to start another circle. Halfway through your reps, reverse direction. Work the other side.

5 Y RAISE

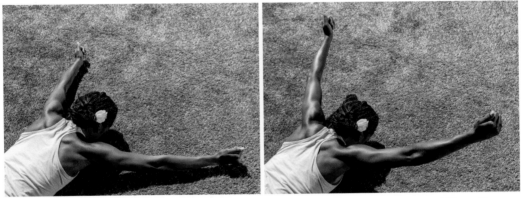

Lie down and squeeze your shoulder blades together to raise and lower your arms in a "Y" position, slow and controlled. Move from your shoulders, with your thumbs leading the way.

RUN

LADDER Run, jog, or walk at the following paces, working your way up and down the ladder:

Long, Slow (RPE 4)	4 minutes	Threshold (RPE 7–8)	2 minutes
Tempo (RPE 6)	3 minutes	Tempo (RPE 6)	3 minutes
Threshold (RPE 7–8)	2 minutes	Long, Slow (RPE 4)	4 minutes
Sprint (RPE 9)	1 minute		

COOLDOWN

▶ Hold each stretch for 5 seconds, take a breath, and see if you can stretch a little farther. Do this 5–6 times, then repeat on the other side.

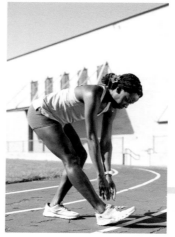

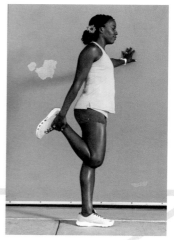

STANDING HAMSTRING STRETCH

Extend one leg just out in front of you and let the knee of the opposite leg bend as you reach forward. Try to keep your back flat.

STANDING QUAD STRETCH

Using a wall for support, stand on one leg and pull the opposite heel to your glute. Press forward through your stretched side to keep your hips and knees square.

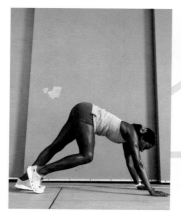

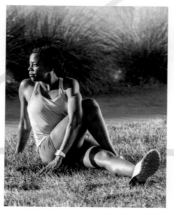

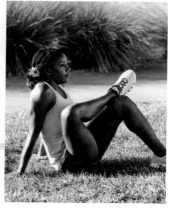

DOWNWARD DOG CALF STRETCH

Push your palms and heels into the ground, bending one knee at a time as you push the opposite heel to the ground to stretch that calf.

SEATED SPINAL ROTATION

With legs extended, cross one leg over the other and twist in the opposite direction, using your arm to push your knee in toward your chest.

SEATED GLUTE STRETCH

With knees bent, cross one leg over the other to get into a figure-4 position. Gently move closer to your stationary foot to intensify the stretch.

TOTAL-BODY STRENGTH + MOBILITY

Pair total-body strength moves with periods of active recovery to keep things interesting and accomplish more in less time. After all, you've got a party to get to!

WARM-UP

▶ Complete an easy 5-minute walk or jog, trying to maintain a consistent pace (RPE 3 to 4) throughout.

ACTIVATION DRILLS

▶ Do 10 reps of each exercise back-to-back with minimal rest.

ROLY-POLY POWER JUMP

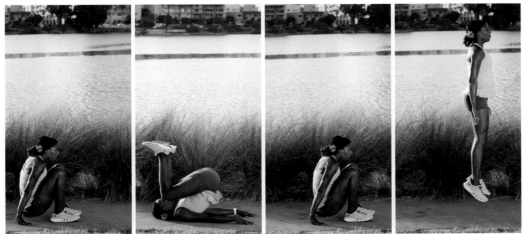

Start in a standing position, sit down, roll backward bringing your knees to chest; then quickly roll up onto your feet and power up into a jump.

BEAR CRAWL

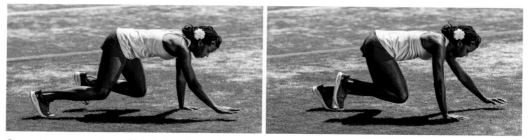

Come to your hands and the balls of your feet, and step forward with one hand and the opposite foot; then step with the opposing hand and foot. Keep your core engaged, back flat, and butt down. Halfway through the reps, move backward.

LATERAL BAND WALK

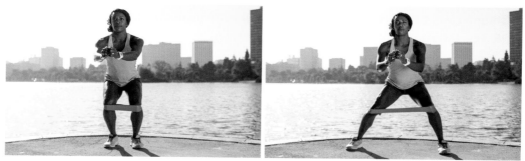

Place a band just below your knees. From a half-squat stance, step one foot out to the side and follow with the opposite foot, keeping the band taut at all times. Return in the opposite direction to work the other side.

DUCK WALK

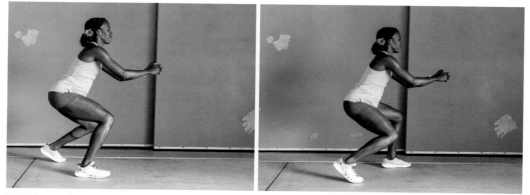

Walk forward in a squat stance, heel first, pushing through the toe. Walk backward, reversing the foot motion, rolling toe to heel.

▶ Each superset begins with a strength exercise, followed by a mobility exercise. Perform 10 to 12 reps of each exercise and repeat for 3 to 4 rounds. Rest for 15 seconds between supersets.

1 WEIGHTED REVERSE LUNGE TO KNEE DRIVE

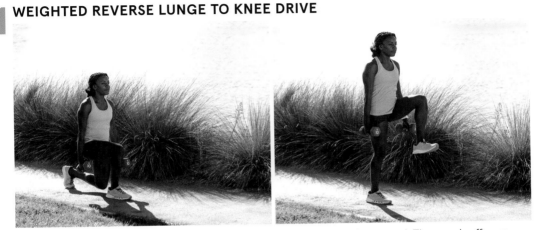

Step back into a lunge, sinking down until your quad is parallel with the ground. Then push off your back foot and bring your knee high before stepping back into a lunge again. Do all of the reps on one side, then switch. Let your legs do the work.

FORWARD LEG SWING

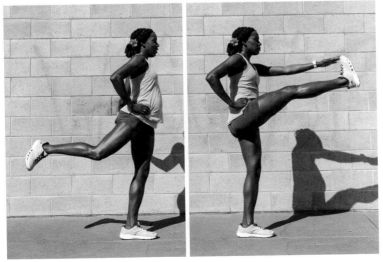

Swing one leg forward and back. Hold a wall for stability if needed. Repeat on the other side.

2 SUMO SQUAT PULSE

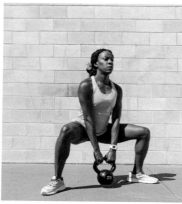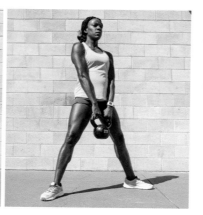

Get into a wide stance with your feet turned out and sink into a squat. Pulse up and down, and let it burn a little.

SIDEWAYS LEG SWING

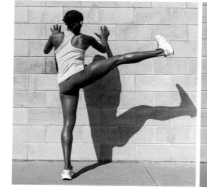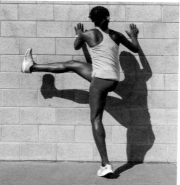

Face the wall and swing one leg from side to side. Work the other side.

3 DEADLIFT TO BENT-OVER ROW

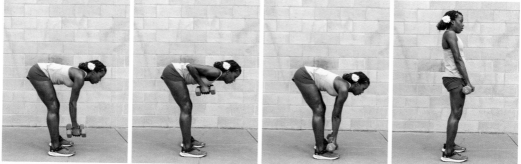

Hinge at the hips and lower the weights close to your body, until your back is parallel with the ground. Turn your palms inwards. Pinch your shoulder blades together as you "row," pulling the weights up to your torso (with elbows tucked); then lower back down. Now push your ribs forward to return to standing.

ACTIVATION

Combining fun running drills and dynamic stretching, this workout will get the blood pumping and promote active mobility.

▶ **Perform each exercise in the superset for 30 seconds and repeat for 3 rounds, resting for 15 seconds between rounds. Rest for 1 minute then start the next superset.**

1 A-SKIP

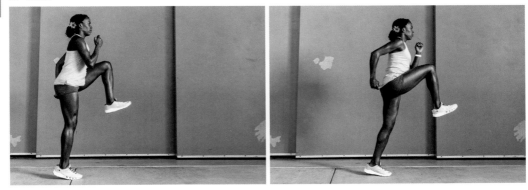

Hop-skip with high knees, swinging your arms to keep momentum.

B-SKIP

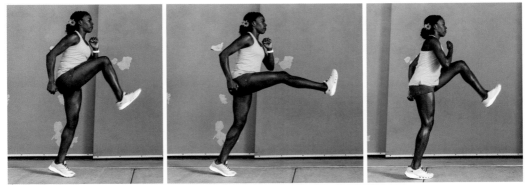

Hop-skip, engaging your glute to pull your knee up (like the A-Skip), then swing your leg forward to extension. Move your arms for momentum.

FORWARD BOUND

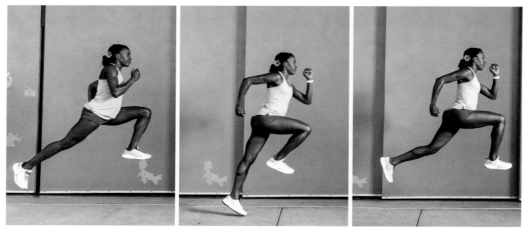

Bound forward, driving off of each foot, and landing soft.

2 SIDE-TO-SIDE HOP-OVER

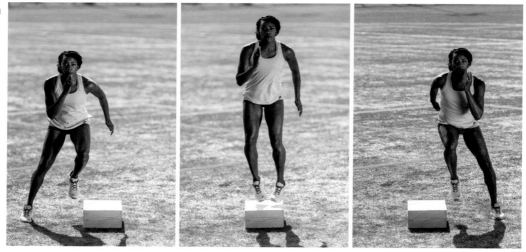

Move from side to side over the top of a step or stationary object, with a quick stutter-step at the top or midpoint. Get your arms pumping opposite your legs for added momentum.

HIGH-KNEE WALL HIKES

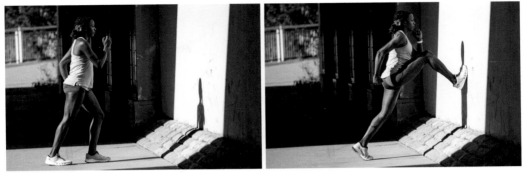

From a staggered stance swing your back leg forward to touch down on the wall as close to hip-height as possible. Swing back to reload, pumping your arms in opposition with your legs. Work both sides.

RUNNING JACK

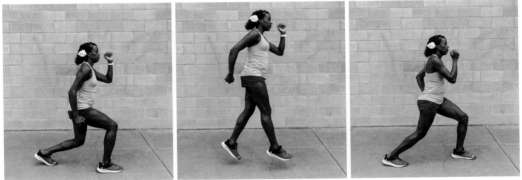

For this jack, jump with one foot forward and one back, arms moving opposite your legs.

SINGLE-LEG POWER-UP

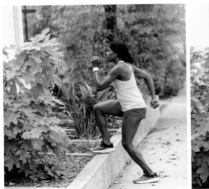

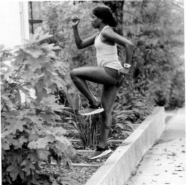

Start with one foot up on a bench or step. Drive through that leg as you explode up and raise your opposite knee toward your chest; then land soft and step back down. Keep a steady rhythm, moving your arms opposite your legs to create momentum. Work both sides.

3 SIDE HURDLE

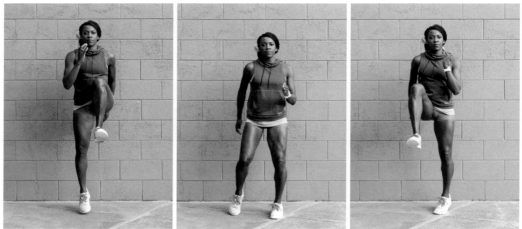

Lift one leg up and step out to the side as if you are stepping over a hurdle, and follow with the trailing leg coming up and over the hurdle. Keep it going, and halfway through the reps, switch direction.

FORWARD LADDER SHUFFLE

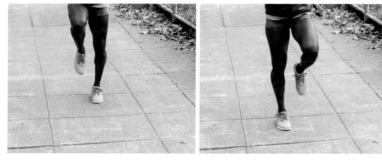

Keeping your feet under your body, spring forward onto one leg, then the other. Move forward with each step as if you're stepping between the rungs of an agility ladder. Pump your arms opposite your fast feet!

LATERAL LADDER

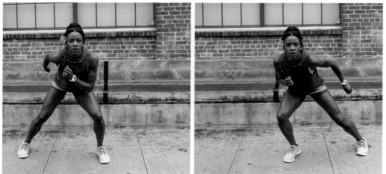

Get in a wide athletic stance and shuffle your feet from side to side, keeping your weight over the inside foot. Pump your arms for momentum and move as quickly as possible. Fast feet!

4 SEATED SPINAL ROTATION

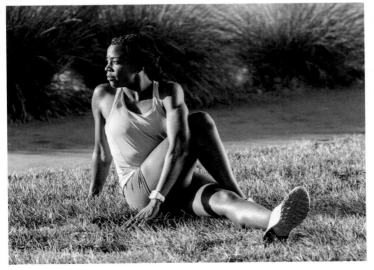

With legs extended, cross one leg over the other and twist in the opposite direction, using your arm to push your knee in toward your chest. Stretch both sides.

HIP SWITCH

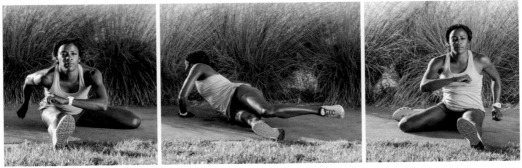

Sit with one leg extended and your other leg bent at a 90-degree angle behind you. Lean forward with the opposite arm leading the stretch. Now swing your back leg around and roll laterally into a stretch on the opposite side. Find your rhythm, moving dynamically from side to side.

▶ Stretch for 5–10 seconds and release. Repeat, maybe taking it a little farther as you exhale. After a few sets, work the other side.

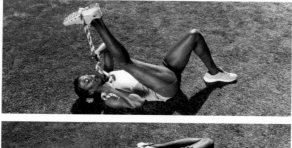

HAMSTRING ROPE STRETCH

Keeping your foot flexed, pull your leg toward your chest. Gently straighten your knee to deepen the stretch.

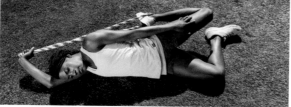

QUAD ROPE STRETCH

Lying on your side, pull your foot toward your butt, keeping it flexed. Let your knee travel behind your hips.

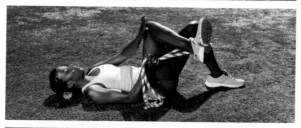

ABDUCTOR ROPE STRETCH

Use the rope to gently pull your foot out to one side, using your hand to keep your knee aligned with your hip.

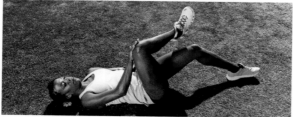

ADDUCTOR ROPE STRETCH

Use the rope to gently pull one foot in toward your torso, using your hand to keep your knee aligned with your hip.

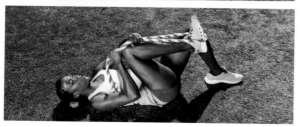

GLUTE ROPE STRETCH

Bring one knee in toward your chest, using the rope to deepen the stretch.

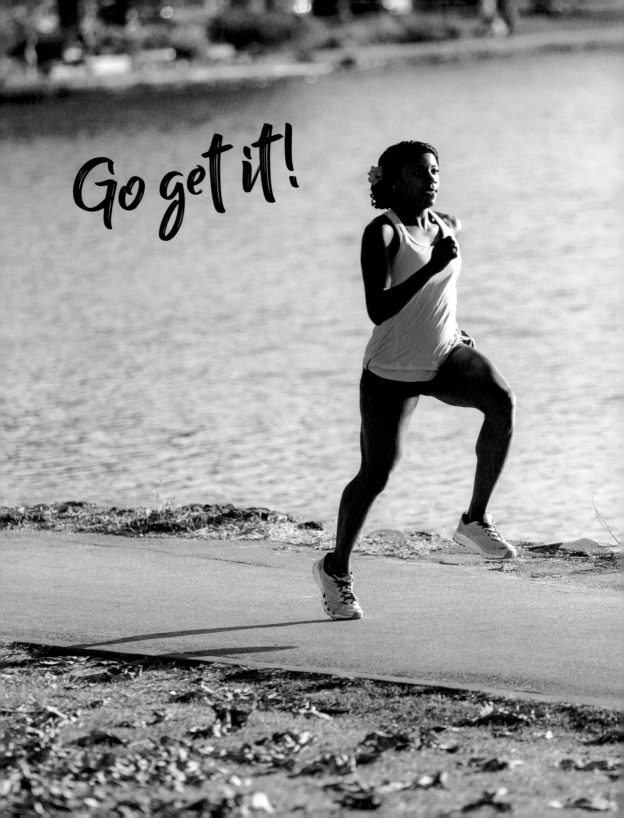

Go get it!

RECOVERY DAYS

If your body needs some rest, give yourself some rest! Mix and match these active recovery ideas to ease tight muscles, recoup your energy, and stay consistent.

FOAM ROLLING ROUTINE

GLUTE ROLL

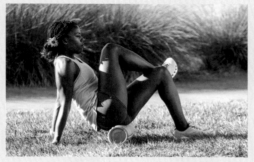

Cross one leg into a figure-4 position and roll out the glute of the stationary leg. Switch sides.

CALF ROLL

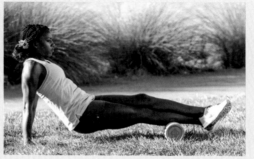

Roll out your calf muscle, using your opposite leg to go a little deeper. Roll out both sides.

UPPER-BACK ROLL

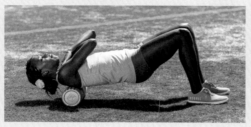

Position a foam roller under your shoulders and lift your hips. Move your feet to shift the roller up and down your back.

HIP FLEXOR ROLL

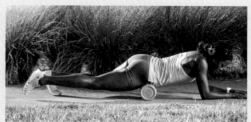

Stabilize yourself with one foot and gently roll out your hip flexor on the opposite leg. Switch sides.

MOBILITY ROUTINE

FORWARD LEG SWING

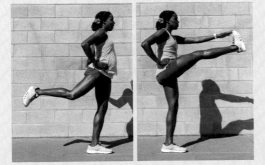

Swing one leg forward and back. Hold a wall for stability if needed. Repeat on the other side.

SIDEWAYS LEG SWING

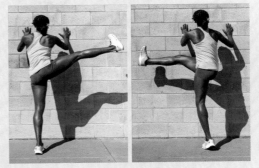

Face the wall and swing one leg from side to side. Work the other side.

HURDLE WALK-OVERS

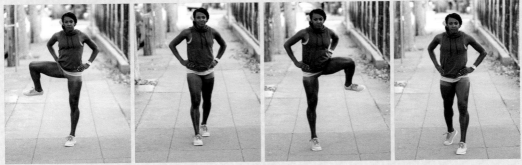

Lift one leg up and out to the side as if you were stepping over a hurdle and moving forward; continue alternating legs.

SIDE HURDLE

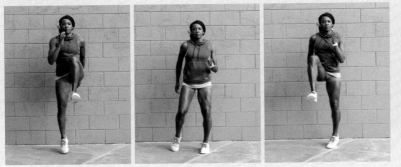

Lift one leg up and step out to the side as if you are stepping over a hurdle, and follow with the trailing leg coming up and over the hurdle. Keep it going, and halfway through the reps, switch direction.

Shout-outs

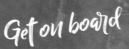

Get on board

#DreamMaternity

Podcasts to fuel your workouts

Keeping-Track

*The Work, Play, Love Podcast
with Lauren & Jesse*

Clean Sport Collective

The Ali on the Run Show

The Humble Sports Podcast

*Simplexity
with Alyson Stoner*

*I'll Have Another with
Lindsey Hein Podcast*

The Running for Real Podcast

*RunGum's
Run The Day Podcast*

C Tolle Run

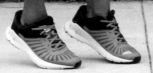

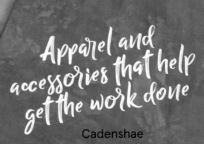

Apparel and accessories that help get the work done

Cadenshae

Altra Running

Nutrition

Nuun Hydration

Picky Bars

Acknowledgments

On the heels of the 2016 Olympic Trials, I received an avalanche of emails from people who watched me tumble and struggle both physically and mentally. I fought, mind, body, and soul, to cross the finish line and face what seemed at face value to be the ultimate disappointment and very sudden end to my lifelong run at Olympic glory. On the other side of it, however, I found myself.

The words of encouragement that I received from complete strangers told me a different story. People recounted the ways I have helped to change the sport; how my passion, desire, and humanness made an impact on them. They talked about the time I ran at USA Nationals in 2015 at eight months pregnant. Women thanked me for using my voice to advocate for women who desire to have both a family and a career. And many people thanked me for speaking out about doping—the abomination that has long plagued the sports world.

Seeing my career through the eyes of others was powerful, like a defibrillator in a moment when I couldn't breathe, like stepping out of quicksand to stand on solid ground. I realized the big picture, what was burning within me, had nothing to do with stepping onto the podium and the shiny things that come with it (though they are pretty cool, too). I found my purpose—who I am, why I do what I do—and why I so boldly, courageously, and unapologetically continue to put one foot in front of the other.

My "Road to Burrito" challenge was born in the aftermath of the Olympic Trials. I put together daily workouts for anyone who needed a little extra motivation to get fit, be better, feel better. I saw it as a way to give a little something back to all of the people who supported me when I most needed that vote of confidence. And this experience was the inspiration for *Feel-Good Fitness*—it's my hope that these challenges will pull you out of your own rough patch or bring you back to a place of confidence.

My children have also shaped my purpose—Linnéa, Aster, and Lennox are beautiful challenges that have been added to my life, shaking up my single-woman routine. It was most noticeable when my daughter and my firstborn, Linnéa, came into this world. She was the one who gave me the gusto to dare to strive for a well-rounded life on my terms. Linnéa was undoubtedly a catalyst for thinking about the world as I wanted it to be presented to her. The challenges I faced—the hardships, the struggles I've known as a woman, as a mom, as someone pursuing big goals—I wanted my daughter to believe that truth, grit, and hard work are the determining factors of success. Linnéa's eyes were the first to bring me back to reality in those moments after crossing that finish line in 2016. She hugged me, loved me unconditionally, and even today she continues to see me as the fastest, smartest, strongest, and bravest woman in the whole world . . . I can't wait until she realizes that *she* is all of those things.

A special thanks to my family: To my mother, who has inspired me to find creative workout routines to fit a busy schedule; to my dad, who was at the forefront of it all, showing me that an active lifestyle is a happy lifestyle; and to my brother, Eric—growing up, he made movement a way of life, play, and fun.

To my husband, Louis, who has without a doubt both supported and enriched my love of movement—we enjoy passing this passion for an active lifestyle on to our children. And to my children, the ones who have given me the opportunity to practice the patience of Mother Teresa, the creativity of Frida Kahlo, and the strength of . . . well, me!

To anyone who is looking to live a healthier, happier, more well-rounded life: It's my hope that you will be patient with the process, creative in the pursuit, and stronger as you take on each new challenge.

About the author

ALYSIA MONTAÑO grew up running the streets, parks, and tracks in and around Los Angeles. Her fleet feet landed her at the University of California, Berkeley, where she proudly represented the Bears as a star middle-distance runner on the track and field team, going on to win six outdoor championships between 2007 and 2015. Alysia took bronze in the 800 meters at the 2010 IAAF World Indoor Championships and picked up another international medal in the 4 × 400 meter relay at the Pan American Games in 2015. She competed for Team USA at the Olympic Games in 2012, finishing fifth in a field riddled with doping allegations that ultimately led to lifetime bans for two of her competitors.

While the sport has handed some hard knocks to Alysia, she has navigated the highs and lows with her relentless sense of humor and radiant optimism, all the while running with a brightly colored flower in her hair and refusing to settle for the status quo. Most recently, she has actively campaigned for changes at the federation level to better address doping in track and field. And having experienced firsthand the challenges that accompany being a professional athlete and starting a family, Alysia has also been an advocate for female athletes to have the financial support needed to compete at the highest level while enjoying a full, healthy life.

Today, Alysia is a working athlete and mom, championing the #DreamMaternity movement together with her cofounder, Molly Dickens, and partners at Cadenshae, Nuun Hydration, and Altra Running, and building &Mother, a nonprofit organization dedicated to breaking down the barriers that limit a woman's choice to pursue and thrive in both career and motherhood. Alysia lives, works, and trains with her husband, Louis, and their three children in Berkeley, California.

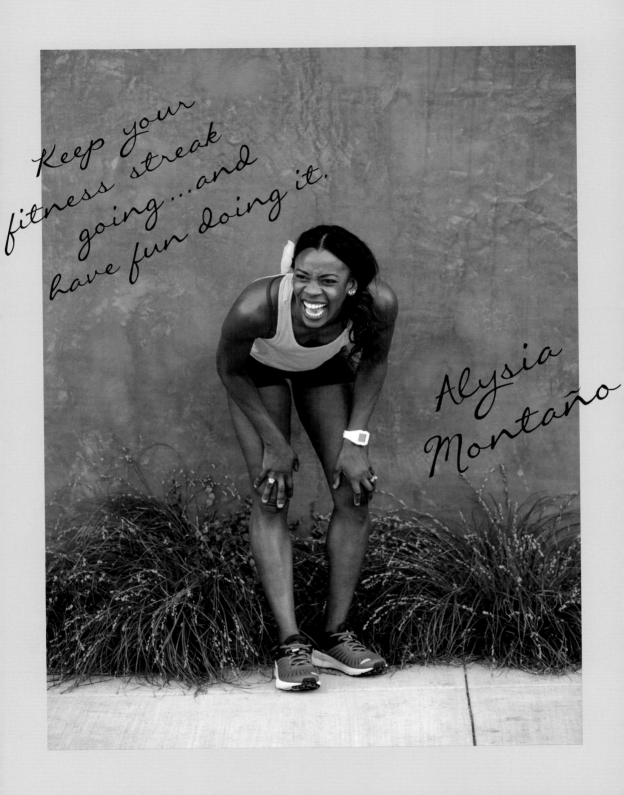

Keep your fitness streak going...and have fun doing it.

Alysia Montaño

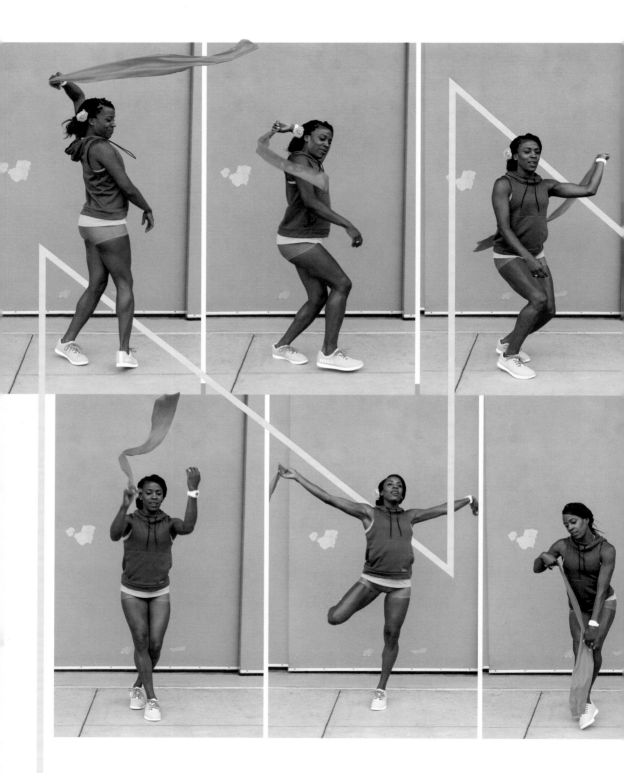

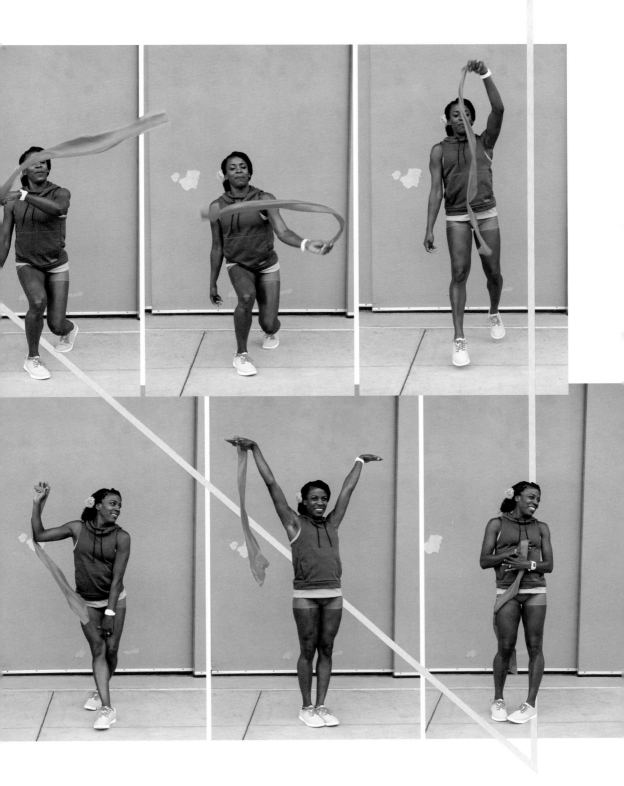

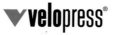